The C. V. Mosby Company
11830 Westline Industrial Drive, St. Louis, Missouri 63141

Library of Congress Cataloging in Publication Data

Helveston, Eugene M   1934-
    Pediatric ophthalmology practice.

    Bibliography: p.
    Includes index.
    1. Pediatric ophthalmology.   I. Ellis, Forrest D.,
joint author.   II. Title.   [DNLM: 1. Eye diseases—In
infancy and childhood.   WW600 H485p]
RE48.2.C5H45   617.7   79-18469
ISBN 0-8016-2129-1

C/CB/B 9 8 7 6 5 4 3 2 1   01/D/078

PEDIATRIC OPHTHALMOLOGY PRACTICE

EUGENE M. HELVESTON, M.D.

Professor of Ophthalmology,
Indiana University School of Medicine,
Indianapolis, Indiana

FORREST D. ELLIS, M.D.

Associate Professor of Ophthalmology,
Indiana University School of Medicine,
Indianapolis, Indiana

with 422 illustrations

The C. V. Mosby Company

ST. LOUIS • TORONTO • LONDON   1980

For the children

Martha

Lisa

Joyce

Kathy

Susan

James

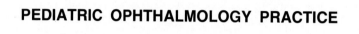

PEDIATRIC OPHTHALMOLOGY PRACTICE

FOREWORD

The average productive career of a physician spans approximately 35 years, which is the time it took ophthalmology's pediatric subspecialty to become viable. In 1944 Costenbader[1] of Washington, D.C., stopped treating adults in order to devote all his time and energy to the ophthalmology needs of infants and children. It was in the same year that Doggart[2] began to write the first text on pediatric ophthalmology, which was published in 1947 by Mosby. Doggart was a general ophthalmic surgeon assigned to the Hospital for Sick Children, Great Ormond Street, London, who perceived a need to acquaint his colleagues with the eye disorders of children. Costenbader was similarly stimulated by what he viewed, while attending at Children's Hospital in his city, to be a need for a more thorough commitment from ophthalmology to focus on pediatric eye problems.

Apparently, the stage was set by the mid 1940s, at least in North America, for the pediatric subspecialty movement to begin among all the recognized specialties in existence at that time. The time was ripe for the advent of pediatric ophthalmology. In fact, the concept of total pediatric care became a veritable magnet that attracted from each specialty a formidable cadre who advanced the pediatric capability of their specialty. As a result, now, every sort of pediatric subspecialty exists, including all the subdivisions of surgery in which ophthalmology is included.

Simultaneous with the development of pediatric ophthalmology was the trend for ophthalmology subspecialization to arbitrarily occur along anatomical and disease-oriented lines (cornea, retina, muscles, lids and orbit, glaucoma, external disease, and so on). Since pediatric ophthalmology is too broad to fit into this pattern, it was viewed by some educators as nonconforming and not in the best interest of ophthalmology. What they overlooked is that subspecialization along anatomical and disease-oriented lines is an intramural

[1]Parks, M. M.: Frank D. Costenbader and the development of pediatric ophthalmology, Children's Hospital National Medical Center 34:101-105, 1978.
[2]Doggart, J. H.: Diseases of children's eyes, St. Louis, 1947, The C. V. Mosby Co.

activity within ophthalmology that lacks the necessary extramural emphasis to relate ophthalmology to the other disciplines of medicine. Pediatric ophthalmology, neuroophthalmology, and ophthalmic pathology relate very well to their counterpart specialties, but to what discipline outside ophthalmology do you relate cornea, muscles, or glaucoma? Obviously, ophthalmology needs both intramural and extramural subspecialization, and gradually this truth became accepted after about 35 years of debate.

Thirty-five years after Doggart, using the same publisher but now with an audience of subspecialists in pediatric ophthalmology, as well as general ophthalmologists and pediatricians, Drs. Helveston and Ellis write on what they perceive to be important, knowledge gained from practicing and teaching exclusively pediatric ophthalmology in middle America. Their intended audience includes both the pediatric ophthalmologist and the general ophthalmologist who, like the family practitioner, must function as a pediatric specialist when serving the needs of a child. Their book updates the information contained in Doggart's text. The balance and evenness of the presentation covering the entire subject is retained by the joint authors of this new text in the same manner as Doggart's text, a feature that is so conspicuously lacking in those texts that comprise a collection of chapters having different authors. Drs. Helveston and Ellis succinctly supply the reader factual material in a concise text containing the necessary illustrations to convey the message.

The authors do not present their work as a strabismus textbook. Ten percent of the total text is devoted to strabismus, providing only the barest coverage of this subspecialty. The current subspecialization pattern tolerates pediatric ophthalmology, an age-related subspecialty, and strabismology, a disease-related subspecialty, to be loosely linked only because the bulk of strabismus occurs in children. In view of this peculiar relationship, the authors are commended for their poise, manifested by keeping the strabismus section in balance with the broader nonstrabismic portion of the text.

Probably for another 35 years a declining number of general ophthalmologists will be practicing part-time pediatric ophthalmology. The guidance that this text will provide them as well as pediatric ophthalmologists makes it a valuable teaching tool that appears just at the time pediatric ophthalmology is beginning the second phase of development. The ramifications of the next developmental phase are now in the realm of interesting speculation. However, one thing is certain: as long as the specialties of pediatrics and ophthalmology exist, the interface between the two always will be pediatric ophthalmology territory.

Marshall M. Parks

PREFACE

The trend in ophthalmology practice in recent years has been toward sub-specialization. Evidence of this is the proliferation of postresidency fellow-ships in the study of the retina, the cornea and external disease, neuroophthal-mology, glaucoma, strabismus and pediatric ophthalmology, and others. These subspecialties are, for the most part, anatomically or disease oriented and, therefore, tend to deal with people of all ages who have a particular type or class of disorder.

Many ophthalmologists in the subspecialty of strabismus have assumed a slightly different role. Because strabismus occurs predominantly in children, a natural "horizontal" spread of the strabismus subspecialist into other areas of children's ophthalmology occurred; hence, the pediatric ophthalmologist. However, a comprehensive study of pediatric ophthalmology turns out to be only slightly less complicated than a study of the entire field of ophthalmolo-gy itself. For this reason, it would be presumptuous to label pediatric ophthal-mology a new subspecialty if it is considered to be free-standing or self-suffi-cient. Perhaps a more appropriate way to think of pediatric ophthalmology is to consider it the subspecialty that deals with the entire spectrum of chil-dren's eye disorders while retaining appropriate interaction with other sub-specialty areas. The pediatric ophthalmologist functions primarily as one who is especially attuned to the needs of children and who is skilled at obtaining information through appropriate history taking and special examination tech-niques. This definition also includes the general ophthalmologist who exam-ines and treats children, because he too is a "pediatric ophthalmologist" when he is dealing with children.

This book is a personal account of our experience in the clinical practice of pediatric ophthalmology. It describes our examination techniques, our expe-riences with some of the more common as well as some of the unusual con-genital and acquired childhood eye diseases, and our treatment plan for some of these conditions. Emphasis is placed on those conditions that are more commonly encountered and for which treatment techniques have been established. No book of this type could be complete nor could it offer in-depth discussion of all conditions that are described. Instead, we intend to provide a "road map" or guide to the physician who deals with eye problems in children. In order to help the reader carry out more complete study, we have included a reading list that we have found useful.

This book is written for the specialist in pediatric ophthalmology, the general ophthalmologist who includes children in his practice, and the pediatrician. Each will use the information in a different way. The specialist in pediatric ophthalmology may compare techniques and use the book as a guide or outline. The general ophthalmologist is given the opportunity to share the point of view of the pediatric ophthalmologist. The pediatrician will be provided information about the function of a child's eyes, methods of examination, pathologic processes, and methods of treatment. Increased awareness by the pediatrician of ocular complications of systemic disease has led to a closer working relationship between the pediatrician and the ophthalmologist. It is hoped that this book will make this cooperative effort more effective for the benefit of the patient.

As pediatric ophthalmology is a cooperative effort, so was this book. We wish to thank Morris Green, M.D., Pediatrician in Chief at James Whitcomb Riley Hospital for Children, Indiana University School of Medicine, for his leadership in assembling an outstanding staff with whom we have worked closely and whom we also thank. The late Frank Costenbader, M.D., laid the groundwork for pediatric ophthalmology, and for this we are all indebted. Marshall M. Parks, M.D., a teacher and friend, has carried on the work started by Dr. Costenbader. Gunter K. von Noorden, M.D., teacher, critic, and friend, has continued his valuable support.

Karen Chevalier-Smith prepared the line drawings, assisted by Craig G. Gosling and his staff. Ken Julian and his staff prepared the photographic material. Bonita Canady, Luelda Carter, Jo Ann Ardery, and Nina Pick provided valuable support. The manuscript was typed by Joanna Emberson with the help of Judy Turpin.

Gopal Krishna, M.D., Chalapathi C. Rao, M.D., and Kenneth A. Haselby, M.D., provided assistance in preparation of Chapter 13, Anesthesia.

Eugene M. Helveston
Forrest D. Ellis

CONTENTS

PEDIATRIC OPHTHALMOLOGY PRACTICE

Chapter 1

VISUAL ACUITY TESTING

Visual acuity testing represents an extremely important part of the practice of pediatric ophthalmology. This testing may be accomplished in a variety of ways, and the results and interpretation of these tests can have far-reaching implications for both the child and his family. Parents may be concerned about whether their child can see normally or perhaps whether he can see at all. Proper immediate treatment, and in some cases long-term expectations and planning, may depend on accurate, early determination of what a child can see. Because this determination must often be made with little "hard" data, especially in the young, the examiner must be skillful and resourceful. Estimates of visual acuity in the very young should be as accurate as possible, but *never* unduly pessimistic.

The determination of visual acuity in infancy can begin as early as the first day of life. Just how well can an infant see? Early studies using an optokinetic drum, which essentially made up the child's entire environment over his crib, indicated that an infant can see at least 20/670. These data were interpreted by some as the limit of the infant's acuity. Actually, these investigators did not use finer optokinetic stripes to test the lower limits of infant acuity, but merely proved that the test could be done on an infant and that infant visual acuity is at least at the stated level. Later examiners showed that as early as the first week of life, an infant can respond to optokinetic stripes, which are comparable to the visual separation found in 20/50 vision.

It is not often that it is critical to determine visual acuity in the neonate, but this does come up occasionally. Concerns about the neonatal problem of retrolental fibroplasia and the increasing tendency toward early surgical intervention for a variety of ocular conditions (including cataract, ptosis, and glaucoma) make information related to visual acuity desirable. In the infant (as with a patient of any age) a reasonable answer should be forthcoming to the question: What can the patient see?

1

In general, visual acuity testing methods in infancy and childhood can be divided into two categories; objective and subjective. *Objective* examination techniques are those that require little or no cooperation on the part of the patient. *Subjective* tests are those that require an interpretation by the patient of what the patient is seeing and the relay of this interpretation back to the examiners. Also, different techniques are required for vision testing of children of different ages. Children may be categorized by age as follows: neonate (birth to 1 month), infant (1 month to 1 year), toddler (1 year to 3 years), preschooler (3 years to 5 years), and schoolager (5 years and up). Each of these categories will be considered individually.

OBJECTIVE METHODS OF DETERMINING VISUAL ACUITY
Affect

Affect involves observation of the individual. This technique is most often used in the very young. Does the infant appear to see or be aware of his surroundings? Does the infant respond to social situations, such as the introduction of the examiner's face or the face of a family member? Does the child look at his own fingers, toes, or objects around his crib? Any recognition of and response to the surroundings should be considered as positive factors in determining that vision is present. Sound or movement that causes reaction to a rush of air across the face or other nonvisual stimuli should be avoided.

Fixation and following

Does the patient steadily fixate on an interesting object? Does he follow interesting objects once eye contact has been made? The following response should be present within the first month or two of life and, of course, is evidence that vision is present.

Ophthalmoscopy

Ophthalmoscopy, both indirect and direct, is useful for determining the clarity of the media and the physical characteristics of the retina and optic nerve. In the presence of clear media and an intact retina with a normal optic nerve, one may assume that the potential for good visual acuity is present unless proved otherwise by other studies.

Pupillary response

The direct and consensual pupillary response to light requires (1) an intact afferent visual pathway to the pregeniculate portion of the optic tract where pupillary fibers synapse in the pretectal area and (2) an intact afferent pathway with third nerve fibers, which, after synapsing at the ciliary ganglion, innervate the pupillary constriction fibers. This light reflex can be considered the *anterior* arc of "vision." The simple maneuver of checking the direct and consensual light reflex tests the anterior half of the visual apparatus but does not indicate that the patient can see. That is, the relay of signals to the cortex and the interpretation of these signals are not tested by a determination of an intact light reflex. If a light shining in one eye produces equal constriction of both pupils, the retina, optic nerve, and optic tract are functioning on the side

2

tested and the pupillomotor fibers of *both* eyes are functioning. If, on the other hand, in the absence of cycloplegic drugs or trauma, shining a light in one eye produces no pupillary constriction in either eye, the first eye, in all likelihood, does not see. If shining a light in the fellow eye produces bilateral pupillary constriction, this confirms that the first eye did not see. A relative afferent defect that produces less pupillary constriction, both direct and consensual, on one side (as determined by moving the light from one eye to the other) indicates an afferent defect and is known as the Marcus-Gunn pupillary phenomenon.

Optokinetic nystagmus

The introduction of an optokinetic instrument, either drum or tape with objects traversing slowly before a normal infant's eyes, will produce an involuntary jerk nystagmus with the fast component in the opposite direction of the movement of the tape or drum. If eye contact has been made with the optokinetic device, the response is involuntary and suggests that vision is present at the cortical level and that the association tracts between cortical vision and the motor nuclei are intact. In general, the finer the stripe or the smaller the target that elicits an optokinetic response, the better the visual acuity. However, it is neither practical nor accurate to grade visual acuity at a meaningful level in an infant by using gradually smaller optokinetic objects.

Anterior and posterior arc of visual response

PLATE 1-1

A Light entering one pupil in a normal individual results in pupillary constriction and confirms an intact anterior arc of visual response as subserved by that eye.

B A repetitive formed stimulus in the form of an optokinetic drum or tape displayed in front of the eyes while the eyes attempt to fixate on the forms passing in front produces an involuntary nystagmus, which confirms an intact posterior visual arc.

C **(1)** Light enters the pupil; **(2)** the light is transmitted through the optic nerve, chiasm, and optic tract; **(3)** the light impulse enters the pretectal area; **(4)** third nerve pupillary constrictor fibers are excited; **(5)** third nerve pupillomotor fibers synapse at the ciliary ganglion; **(6)** pupillary constrictor fibers are activated, resulting in pupillary constriction; **(7)** the light impulse synapses at the lateral geniculate; **(8)** light impulses are received at the occipital cortex. Through association fibers in the brain, the oculomotor nuclei are stimulated, and impulses are sent to the eye muscles, producing optokinetic nystagmus, which confirms that the posterior visual arc is intact and that the individual tested can see the objects presented in the optokinetic target.

4

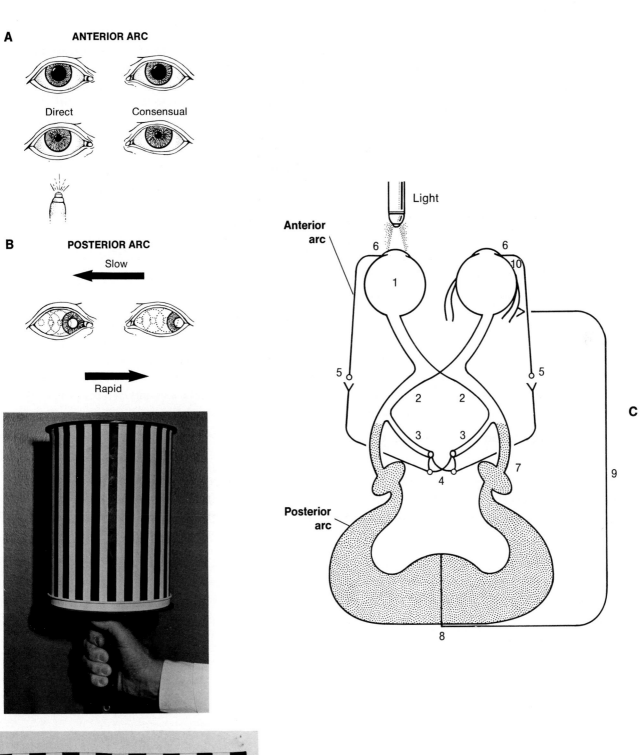

A ANTERIOR ARC

Direct   Consensual

B POSTERIOR ARC

Slow

Rapid

Light

Anterior
arc

Posterior
arc

C

PLATE 1-1

5

Visually evoked response (Plate 1-2, A)

Visually evoked response (VER) is determined by stimulating the eyes with a bright flash while recording electrical activity through scalp electrodes placed over the visual cortex. It is, in essence, a focal electroencephalogram. This test can be useful in confirming cortical blindness in infants and young children. It has little value as a quantitative determination. In a child with suspected cortical blindness but with a normal retina and an intact pupillary response and questionable optokinetic nystagmus (OKN) response, an absent VER confirms cortical blindness. Probably the most valuable place for this test is in the mentally retarded individual who acts blind but who has a normal fundus. In such a case, when a normal VER is found, the apparent blindness may be attributed to an intellectual deficit. A *relative* difference in the VER occurs in functional amblyopia when patterned stimuli are used and amplitude is measured. The amblyopic eye produces a lower amplitude cortical response. Defects such as optic atrophy may produce a delay between stimulus and cortical response.

Electroretinogram (Plate 1-2, B)

An electroretinogram (ERG) measures the electrical response of the retina to flashing lights. Children who have evidence of Leber's amaurosis, tapetoretinal degeneration, or a family history of retinitis pigmentosa or other retinopathies require an ERG. This is not really a vision test but is rather a test of retinal function, which may be necessary to localize a visual defect to the retina or to define the nature of the defect.

Electrooculogram (Plate 1-2, C)

An electrooculogram (EOG) measures the electrical potential between the back and the front of the eye as the eyes move from side to side. This test is useful primarily as a method of confirming vitelliruptive macular degeneration. Other family members who carry the defective gene but who are unaffected clinically will have a reduced or abnormal EOG. The EOG does not indicate visual acuity and cannot be done accurately in the absence of useful vision. A reduced or absent ERG obviates the need for or the ability to interpret the EOG.

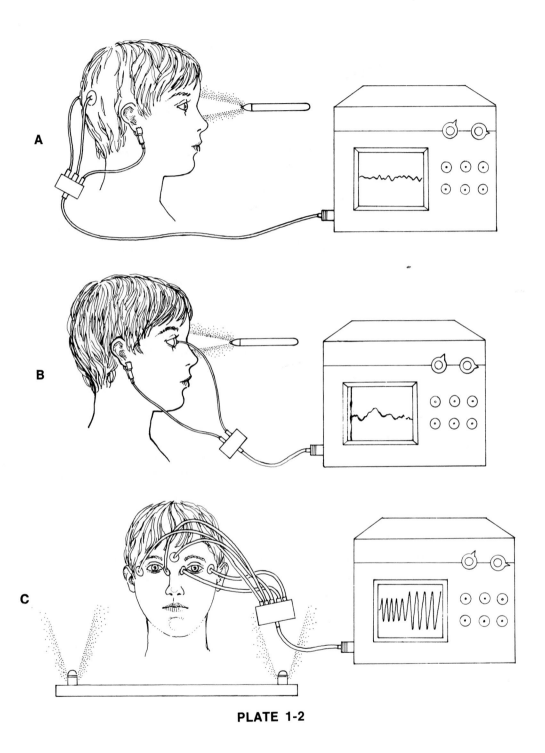

PLATE 1-2

Visuscope examination

This test, although primarily objective, does require that the patient attempt to look at the fixation target, and therefore requires cooperation on the part of the patient. Eccentric fixation is synonymous with poor vision. Eccentric fixation usually occurs in one eye only and usually is the sequela of functional amblyopia. The test is performed by projecting a fixation object on the retina and asking the patient to look directly at the object. If a retinal area other than the fovea is chosen for fixation, vision in that eye will be reduced. In general, the farther from the fovea that fixation occurs, the less steady fixation will be and the poorer vision will be.

SUBJECTIVE TESTS FOR DETERMINING VISUAL ACUITY
Finding objects

In toddlers, a useful subjective visual acuity test can be accomplished by silently placing interesting objects around the room, and then asking the child to locate and retrieve these objects. A coin tossed onto the floor as the child watches will be readily retrieved by an alert youngster with useful vision. If the child has enough intelligence and vision to recognize sample objects shown him and understands that he is free to locate them, some useful information can be obtained. This test is a help in demonstrating the presence of visual capabilities to the parents. This finding of objects is used mostly for children of toddler to preschool age who have visual acuity in the neighborhood of 20/200 or better as determined by other means.

Optotype recognition (Plate 1-3)

Allen cards are pictures that can be useful as the first subjective visual acuity test in a child between 2½ and 3½ years of age. Allen cards ordinarily present only a single optotype; therefore, the crowding phenomenon is not present, and, in the case of functional amblyopia, visual acuity may be recorded erroneously as being better than it actually exists under usual seeing circumstances. Visual acuity testing with Allen cards is done at a 10-foot distance using a 20/30 optotype. Therefore, the acuity level is recorded as 10/30, or, if the acuity is poor, the cards are moved closer to the child, and the acuity is recorded as 8/30, 5/30, and so on. Allen card testing and isolated E testing produce similar results. Allen card testing should be used only in children who are unable to cooperate for more sophisticated tests, such as the linear illiterate E or the alphabet.

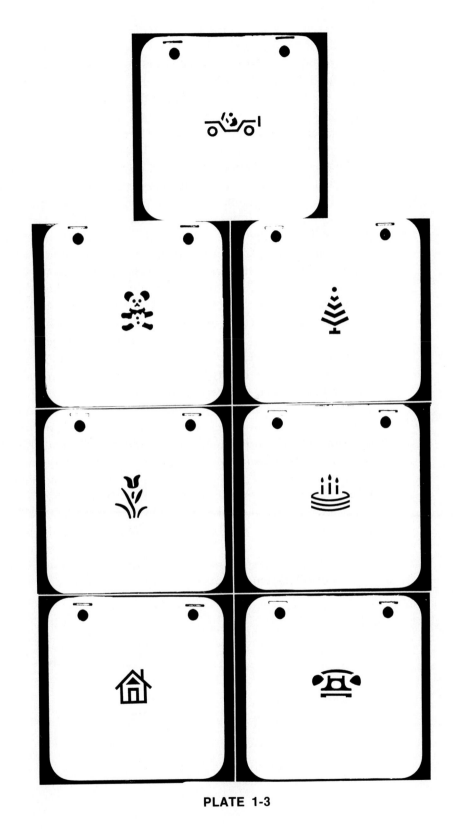

PLATE 1-3

Illiterate E (Plate 1-4)

Illiterate E testing is carried out with a full chart. Any cooperating child of normal intelligence and sufficient age should be able to perform this test after a few seconds of instruction. The youngest age for linear E testing usually is age 3 for girls and 3½ for boys. We ordinarily have the patient use his hand to mimic the direction of the fingers of the E on the chart, or the child may be given a cutout E to mimic the direction of the optotype. The technique we employ for the illiterate E vision test is to have the child observe the initial optotype (E) in progressively smaller lines until he makes an error. The examiner then tests across the lowest line on which the child correctly identifies the initial optotype. If, while reading across any line, the patient recognizes more than half of the optotypes, he is credited as responding to that line, with notation made of the number of minuses for the missed optotypes, such as 20/30−2. If more than half of the optotypes are missed, the patient is credited for the lowest complete line seen and is given credit for extra optotypes seen, such as 20/40+2. If the patient responds correctly to the entire line, another attempt is made at having him see the line below. When the best acuity is obtained in the first eye checked (usually the right), it is occluded and the acuity is checked in the fellow eye. A known amblyopic eye is tested first. Testing of the fellow eye begins at the lowest line that could be seen by the first eye tested. If the second eye cannot perform at this level, the examiner moves up to successively larger optotypes until the patient succeeds. Then vision is checked across that line proceeding from right to left. This technique allows the examiner to obtain the maximum amount of information with the minimum potential for fatiguing or losing the interest of the child. The final acuity determination should be made with a *horizontal* line of optotypes, because in cases of functional amblyopia, single or isolated optotypes of a given size can be seen more readily than the same size optotype presented with a similar visual target on either side. This crowding phenomenon is frequently present in cases of functional amblyopia. Often, a child will get the first and last letters correct on a line, but will be unable to correctly identify the central letters for the next several lines. In this instance, vision should be recorded as best full-line acuity and as best acuity with crowding. An example could be: OD 20/50 (full-line), 20/25 (crowding).

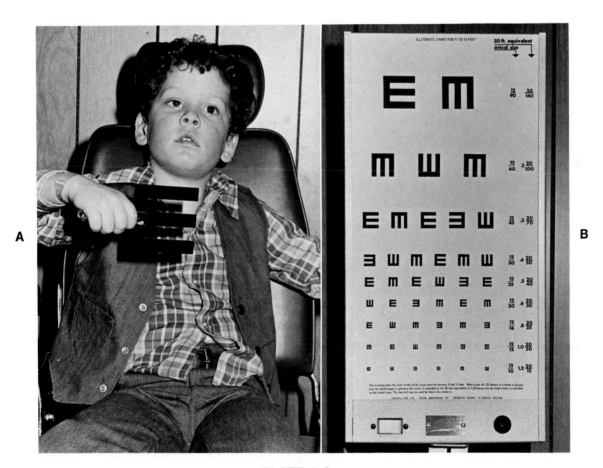

A   B

PLATE 1-4

11

The alphabet (Plate 1-5)

In the late preschool-age child or in the school-age child, visual acuity testing is done with the usual Snellen chart. Whole lines should be presented because of the crowding phenomenon. A projected chart or a self-illuminated chart may be employed. Vision is recorded as with the illiterate E. The Stycar and similar matching vision tests utilize a matching set of symbols, which the child selects to indicate his interpretation of the distance symbol. These types of tests eliminate part of the abstract requirements of the Snellen chart.

Near vision

It is important to check near vision at least in children who can read, and occasionally it is useful to check near vision in the preschool nonreader. The most useful way to check near vision is to ask the patient to read a paragraph. This acts both as a visual acuity test and as a reading test (see Chapter 14). In the nonreading child, numbers or Es may be used for the near vision test.

Color vision testing

Color vision testing may not be done unless a retinal dystrophy is suspected, the family history is positive, or the family specifically requests it. Eight percent of white males have some red-green color deficiency, whereas only ½% to 1% of females are affected. In isolation, this defect rarely results in any real drawback to normal function, especially in childhood. We think that no special emphasis should be placed on the diagnosis of "color blindness" at early childhood examination. Although the identification of such defects can be helpful in a classroom situation, too much emphasis must not be placed on these minor abnormalities at this age. A diagnosis of "color blindness" may unnecessarily limit the activities of an individual through misguided redirection of future job selection. Tritanopia, or blue-yellow "color blindness," is estimated to occur in 0.0001% of individuals. This does not represent a clinically significant entity. American blacks and Orientals have approximately one-half the incidence of red-green color blindness that Caucasian males have. When color vision is tested, an Ishihara test or an AO H-R-R booklet is used, and the patient is asked to respond, identifying the numbers or patterns. A specific diagnosis can be made by comparing the pattern or response with a key in the testing booklet. For older children, the Farnsworth-15 and 100-hue tests may be used, as well as the Nagel anomaloscope.

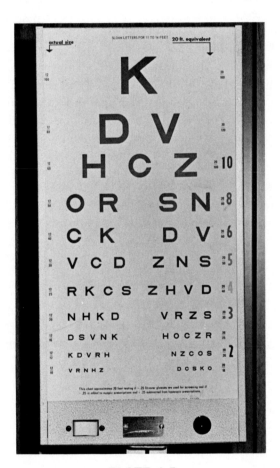

PLATE 1-5

13

VISUAL ACUITY DETERMINATION BY AGE
Visual acuity determination in the neonate (birth to 1 month)
(Plate 1-6, A)

Visual acuity in the neonate is interpreted by objective means. Objective evidence of clear media and an intact retina should be established using the direct and indirect ophthalmoscope and the retinoscope. A persistent pupillary membrane or tunica vasculosa lentis may be present. These usually disappear completely, or a small vestige that is of no clinical significance will remain. In the premature infant, transient lens opacities may be present. These usually disappear within a few weeks. If the media are clear, the retina is intact, and no inequality in retinoscopy exists, it is probable that the child will have good vision. This type of examination should include determination of the pupillary reactions. Response to the OKN tape or drum and a blink response to a threatening gesture indicate that cortical reception of visual stimuli is present. An infant should show some interest in following large objects in his environment by the age of 1 to 2 months. It is an important rule of thumb in such examinations to remain optimistic rather than pessimistic with regard to the final level of visual acuity. Unless a severe structural abnormality is found, such as a coloboma, cataract, hypoplastic nerve, unilateral high myopia, or persistent hyperplastic vitreous, the parents should be advised to assume a "wait and see" attitude. Without unnecessarily or unfairly developing false expectations, the examiner should allow the parents to retain realistic optimism with regard to their infant's visual future.

VISUAL ACUITY ACCORDING TO AGE

Age	Acuity	Method of testing
Neonate (Birth to 1 month)	20/50 – 20/100	*Objective* Observe OKN

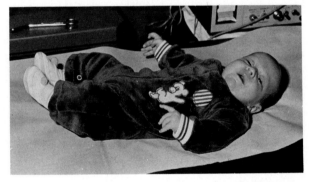

PLATE 1-6

Visual acuity testing in the infant (1 to 12 months) (Plate 1-6, B)

Objective determination of the media and the retina, using retinoscopy, is carried out as noted above. As with the neonate, a great deal of information can be obtained from this examination. Retinoscopy becomes easier when the patient is about 6 months old. In certain selected indications, glasses may need to be prescribed at this early age. Occasional cases of refractive accommodative esotropia occur before 1 year of age. Also, unilateral high myopia is best treated if detected and optically corrected early. The visual examination of the patient continues with an evaluation of the child's awareness of his surroundings. During infancy, the child should be very much aware of his surroundings and should respond appropriately to social situations. It is important to bring stimulating objects into the infant's line of sight silently. Children are adept at following sounds, and it is important to differentiate between response to a sound and the following of an object because of visual interest. Pupillary reactions (both direct and consensual) are determined, as well as a blink response to a threatening gesture. An OKN drum or tape can be used effectively in this age group. The optokinetic stimulus should be presented horizontally from both the right and left and vertically both up and down. If congenital nystagmus has been noted, one may observe that the horizontal component can be converted to a vertical component by OKN stripes or targets. This patient would be expected to have a final visual acuity of better than 20/200, possibly approaching normal visual acuity. The child's fixation behavior can be determined fairly accurately during the first year of life. If the child habitually fixates with one eye and cannot be made to fixate with the other eye, it is certain that visual acuity is poor in the nonfixating eye. This may be on the basis of a functional or an organic defect. In some instances, this test may be difficult to interpret because most infants object to having either eye occluded, regardless of whether it is the better seeing eye or not. In cases where the child actually uses his hand to push the occluder away when it occludes one of his eyes while not objecting to occlusion of the other eye, the examiner should have a strong suspicion that extremely poor vision is present in the nonpreferred eye. In our experience, such response has been more often associated with organic defects such as optic atrophy, colobomas, cataract, and persistent hyperplastic primary vitreous, rather than functional amblyopia. In cases of strabismus, the observation of habitual fixation with one eye suggests a diagnosis of amblyopia. In cases of suspected cortical blindness, results of the VER test can be of some value. If any indication of sight is obtained by the above examinations, however, the VER probably will not reveal any new useful information. In our experience, the VER has been useful in a clinical sense only in providing objective evidence that cortical blindness is either present or not present.

16

VISUAL ACUITY ACCORDING TO AGE (cont'd)

Age	Acuity	Method of testing
Infant (1 month to 12 months)	20/50+	*Objective* Observe OKN VER

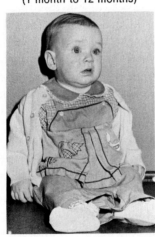

PLATE 1-6, cont'd

Visual acuity determination in the toddler (1 to 3 years) (Plate 1-7, A)

The objective examination is carried out by observing the child's awareness of his surroundings, pupillary reactions, and the OKN responses. In the toddler age group, response to alternate occlusion can be more meaningful than in infants. Chronic fixation with one eye accompanied by objection to occlusion of this eye is strong evidence that poor vision and possibly an organic defect or amblyopia exist in the fellow eye. As in the infant, strong preference for one eye in the presence of clear media and in the absence of a pathologic fundus condition is an indication for occlusion of the preferred eye because of presumed functional amblyopia in the nonpreferred eye. Coins or other similar-sized objects may be placed quietly on a carpeted surface while the patient is being observed while he is not looking, then the child who can walk can be asked to find these small objects. This test, carried out in the presence of the parents, provides objective evidence that some vision is present and provides encouragement to parents that their child can see small objects.

It is not uncommon to examine a child who later turns out to have visual acuity of only 20/200 or less whose parents say that he can pick up the tiniest objects off the floor at home. We are primarily interested in how a child can function in the world in which he must live. For this reason, optimism and realistic expectations should be combined. Severely affected children, such as those with advanced retrolental fibroplasia, large colobomas, or dense corneal or lenticular opacities, will be especially fascinated by shafts of light coming through venetian blinds or window shades and shining on the floor. Persistent fascination with these types of stimuli may be an indication that visual acuity is very poor. Parents often are unduly impressed and optimistic about such behavior.

During the toddler years, parents may realize for the first time that they have a truly "blind" or severely visually handicapped child. While this reality is sinking in to the parents, it is important for the physician to be both supportive and realistic. Parents should be shown what the child can do more than what he cannot do, but at the same time parents should be urged to seek the best possible advice for obtaining an effective education for the child. Most state agencies for the blind have counselors who will assist families in planning for the rearing of a blind or visually deprived child. The ophthalmologist should now restrain the overly optimistic parents and buoy up the overly pessimistic parents.

Allen cards that contain outlines of familiar figures can be a useful method for determining visual acuity in toddlers. These cards depict such objects as a car, Christmas tree, teddy bear, birthday cake, telephone, horse and rider, and a flower. These objects are designed for use at distances of 10 feet and less. Best visual acuity is usually recorded as 10/30. If the child cannot identify the card at 10 feet, it is moved closer to him, and the notation may be 5/30, 2/30, and so on. Use of the Allen cards with a single optotype does not take into consideration the crowding phenomenon. However, the more intricate composition of some of these objects may in part negate this defect. A VER may be used with toddlers but has been employed very infrequently by us to provide reproducible data confirming cortical blindness. With regard to amblyopia in toddlers, the most important factor is equality of visual acuity. It is of no real benefit to determine if a toddler has better than 10/30 (20/60) visual acuity in *each* eye. This will probably become normal vision, 20/20, during the maturing process. On the other hand, a *difference* in visual acuity is very significant in this age group. For example, if a child sees 10/30 with the right eye and 6/30 with the left, the serious possibility exists that functional amblyopia is present in the left eye. This difference in visual acuity demands treatment. During this period, any anisometropia over 1 to 1½ D sph or cyl should be considered for correction. The timely use of correcting glasses eliminates or greatly reduces the likelihood of the development of microtropia, monofixation syndrome, or anisometropic amblyopia.

Visual acuity testing in the preschool years (3 to 5) (Plate 1-7, B)

Objective methods are continued. These include evaluation of the media, retinoscopy, and evaluation of the retina (see p. 2).

Response is determined as the patient's awareness of his surroundings. Pupillary reactions, both indirect and direct, and optokinetic response may be done. If strabismus is present, note should be made of the preferred eye. If alternation of fixation is noted, amblyopia can be ruled out. The degree of preference for one eye can be a rough measure of the depth of amblyopia; that is, the more a given eye is preferred, the greater the amblyopia in the fellow eye. The preschool child may be asked to find small objects on the floor, and Allen cards can be used for single optotype determination. However, most children in this age group who have at least average intelligence can be responding with an E chart. Girls 3 years old and boys 3½ years old should be able to respond to the Es readily. Our practice is to give just a few seconds' instruction in use of the E chart for such children. If they are able to understand and cooperate in this brief instruction period, the examination is carried out. If they do not understand the E game after 1 minute or so of explanation, our experience has shown that further instruction on that day will not be fruitful, and other testing methods should be used. If the E chart testing is not successful, the child is tested with the Allen cards and his parents are advised to teach the E game at home. Many children are able to cooperate with the letter chart during the preschool years. Our scheme for determination of both E chart and letter visual acuity is a simple one that makes the most of the child's attention span in order to obtain the most meaningful test results. The left eye is occluded, and the child is asked to identify the first symbol of each line. When he misses a symbol, the examiner moves up to the smallest line that the patient could identify, and visual acuity is tested across that line. The occluder is changed to the other eye, and the patient is asked to read the same line, this time from right to left. If the patient correctly identifies the initial optotype on this line, the next smaller symbol down is tested. If the patient responds correctly, the examiner points out increasingly smaller symbols at the end of each line. When the child fails a symbol, the examiner moves back up to the smallest line in which a correct answer was given and the line is checked from right to left. This enables the child to report the best possible visual acuity with the minimum number of responses being required.

It is an exercise in futility to ask a child to read every letter on the chart. Certain children have only a given number of responses in them for a given day. Regardless of whether he can see the object or not, the child stops responding when he becomes tired or is bored with the game.

Stereoacuity testing is valuable in the preschool age group. A child who has good stereoacuity probably has good visual acuity. A stereoscopic response of nine out of nine Titmus dots or 40 sec of arc disparity indicates that visual acuity is at least 20/40 in the poorer eye and, of course, indicates the presence of good binocular cooperation.

We do color vision testing only in a superficial way, as indicated previously. We avoid assigning any undue importance to color vision testing, except in cases of achromatopsia or in cases where color vision testing is important as a retinal function test. In such cases, visual acuity will be reduced, and the need for color testing will be apparent at the time of the examination. In cases of achromatopsia, or absence of color vision, visual acuity is always 20/200 or less and nystagmus is present.

Any child in the amblyopia-susceptible years should be checked more for equality of vision than for absolute visual acuity. That is, a visual acuity of 20/30 OD and 20/60 OS is far less acceptable than visual acuity of 20/40 in each eye. Even visual acuity of 20/50 in each eye may be acceptable. Bilaterally reduced visual acuity is more likely to end up as good binocular visual acuity when the child matures than is unequal visual acuity with two lines or more of difference between the two eyes, even when the better eye is 20/20 or 20/30. The wearing of proper glasses and, when needed, carefully supervised patching, should be carried out in all cases of amblyopia in childhood.

Vision testing in the school-age patient (Plate 1-7, C)

If no other indication for an eye examination exists, we think that it is important for each child to have an accurate visual acuity test before starting school. This should be done preferably between the ages of 3½ and 5 years. The Snellen alphabet chart is used in the distance, and paragraph reading is used at near. When abnormalities in vision are found, any appropriate treatment should then be carried out. After the child enters school, school vision testing done in the third, fifth, and eighth grades is ordinarily satisfactory. Myopia usually calls attention to itself, and usually does not represent a serious academic handicap over the short term. Hyperopia, provided it does not cause a refractive esotropia, is of no real significance unless it is of such a great degree that bilateral ametropic amblyopia or asthenopia symptoms result. Symmetrical, with the rule, astigmatism also is a relatively benign condition that may cause only slight reduction in visual acuity and that may escape notice until the child is older.

Color vision testing may be carried out in special instances for the reasons stated previously.

There is a great deal of misinformation among the lay public regarding

20

VISUAL ACUITY ACCORDING TO AGE (cont'd)

	Age	Acuity	Method of testing

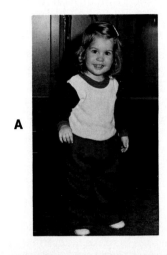

A

Toddler
(1 year to 3 years)

20/40 +

Objective and subjective
Observe   Allen cards
OKN   "E" game
VER   Find objects
ERG

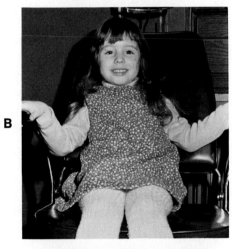

B

Preschool
(3 years to 5 years)

20/30 +

Subjective
Allen cards
"E" game
Alphabet

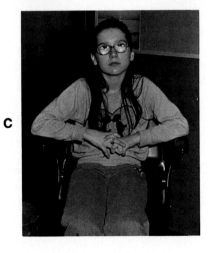

C

School age
(5 years to 16 years)

20/16

Subjective
Alphabet

PLATE 1-7

color vision. A recent example of misguided zeal was brought to our attention. Investigators found a surprisingly high proportion of blue/yellow color blindness (13%) in a group of 3-year-olds tested with the Muncel 15-hue color test. The researchers suggested blue/yellow color blindness as a reason for poor performance with blue mimeographed handout sheets in school. However, when this test was repeated in 3-year-olds by other researchers, who had the children arrange the colors beginning with the blue end of the spectrum and ending at the red, no cases of blue/yellow color blindness were found. The second investigators inferred that a fatigue factor resulted in the erroneous diagnosis of color blindness to blue that was found by the original researchers. Unfortunately, correcting damage done by an erroneous test is not an easy task.

Visual field testing

Accurate central or peripheral visual field testing can ordinarily be done on a cooperative child of 7 or 8, but only occasionally before that age. About the best that can be done in a child under this age is to make an estimate of the visual field by the confrontation technique. To do this, the examiner faces the patient and closes his own left eye and occludes the patient's right eye. Fingers, a light, or another object is brought from the periphery while the examiner sees that the patient maintains fixation on the examiner's eye. The examiner asks the patient to count the fingers or identify the object presented when he sees the object come into view from the visual periphery. The examiner compares his field in each eye with that of the patient. Field defects can be detected with reliability in this manner, but congruity can only be estimated.

VISION SCREENING

Vision screening in the preschool years can be carried out by a variety of techniques. Most pediatricians or family physicians make some type of vision test available to their patients. The accuracy of such tests depends as much on the training and interest level of the individual administering the test as on the patient. Organizations such as the National Society for the Prevention of Blindness have established standards for the performance of preschool vision testing. Carried out on the state level, mass preschool vision screening is provided by local societies according to criteria established by the national society. Such vision screening is done using the linear E. Although standards vary from state to state, referral to an eye doctor is usually made if the visual acuity in the poorer eye is 20/40 or less or if two or more lines of difference between the two eyes exist. The effectiveness of such screening depends on the establishment of local volunteer societies and the compliance of the families in making their children available for screening examination. After screening, appropriate referral should be initiated and followed up. In spite of attempts to reach all testable children and to have all referrals carried out, the society's diligent efforts have fallen far short of the goal that all children be screened.

A recently promoted *home eye test* is being sponsored by the National Society for the Prevention of Blindness. This test can be requested by contacting the society's headquarters. Detailed instructions are included with the test, which allows the family to administer the eye test to individual children. The results are interpreted by the family, who are instructed to either pass or fail the child. If failure is noted and reported to the society, appropriate measures with regard to further examinations are suggested. A trial of this test done by us indicated that the false negative rate was approximately equal to the incidence of amblyopia found in a general population; that is, in the neighborhood of 2% to 3%. This raised the concern that such a home-administered test, done without proper supervision, could result in the well-intended but misguided overlooking of a large percentage of patients with amblyopia.

Other home eye tests have been proposed, such as a home television screener. This type of examination certainly holds promise for the future.

Some states require that a vision test be completed before a child enters school. Other states perform vision testing as part of the entry process into school. At the present time, no uniform program exists for preschool vision screening.

Levels of visual impairment

It is useful to have certain functional guideposts with regard to visual acuity levels. An arbitrary but useful scheme explaining what type of activities an individual can be expected to engage in successfully may contain eight basic levels as follows.

Normal vision with binocularity

If a patient has 20/20 vision in each eye and normal stereoacuity to 40 sec of arc disparity, he has normal vision. In the absence of color blindness, excessive phorias or significant refractive error, or ocular disease, he is considered to have "perfect" vision. With a corrected refractive error or a large phoria, he could be considered to have functionally normal eyes, albeit with the correctable abnormality. These abnormalities are significant only if a person attempts to pass a certain rigorous eye test, such as one required for commercial or military aviation or astronaut training.

Normal vision

If an individual has visual acuity of 20/20 in each eye, distance and near, with or without correction, his *vision* is said to be normal. Twenty-twenty vision may exist in a patient with strabismus and a functional loss of vision at any given time in the nonfixing eye. People with 20/20 vision, even in the presence of strabismus, have little meaningful impairment of their ability to function except for the reduction in stereopsis and reduced peripheral fields, in the case of larger angles of esotropia. This, of course, is the case in a patient whose sensorial adaptations have eliminated diplopia.

Driver's license vision

If an individual can see between 20/60 and 20/70 in his best corrected eye, he will be able to obtain a driver's license, although possibly with some restrictions. It is important practically and psychologically for teenagers to be able to reach this level of acuity. The increased mobility and independence associated with being able to drive is of immeasurable importance.

School vision

With visual acuity between 20/70 and 20/200, an individual should be able to obtain an education in the usual public school setting with the use of normal-sized print. Near vision is almost always better than distance vision, and with the use of magnifiers or a high plus bifocal, a person who is properly motivated should be able to attend the usual school setting with his peers if his teachers are attuned to his problem. Special education classes are now available in most schools to offer additional help to the handicapped student.

Legal blindness (20/200)

If a person has visual acuity of 20/200 or less, and/or a visual field of 20° or less in the better eye, he is legally blind. This is of use only as a legal definition. It allows special considerations with regard to taxes, entrance into special schools, eligibility for aid, and other arbitrarily arrived-at "benefits." Legal blindness should not be interpreted as a medical term and should not become of itself a barrier to functioning in the most productive way. The term should not be used to describe the vision in one eye when the fellow eye has better vision than 20/200, nor should it be used to describe uncorrected ametropia.

Travel vision

Visual acuity of 20/400± will allow the individual to travel in unfamiliar surroundings provided he is otherwise healthy. The use of print may be possible but difficult. Special education, probably with learning Braille, may be required; however, an unsheltered educational experience may be accomplished by the highly motivated individual who has some extra help.

Light perception

Light perception is primarily important for the individual's sense of well-being and may be an aid in mobility, but is not useful for other educational purposes.

No light perception

This, of course, is the "end of the line," and the diagnosis is determined only after exhausting all possibilities that the patient can possibly see.

School for the blind

Most states have one or more schools for the blind. These are usually residential schools and in most instances contain children who have severe visual handicaps of well below 20/200. However, there has been some change in eligibility determination in recent years. Federal laws have mandated local school systems to provide education for handicapped children, including the blind. In addition, schools for the blind have been required to provide education for children with emotional disturbances and retardation. Therefore, schools for the blind have been changed in character and now educate the multiply handicapped as well as the blind. If education in a school for the blind is contemplated, it is important that the family, child, and authorities at the school for the blind be acquainted early. It is important for a child entering the blind school environment to be well prepared for this experience.

In many instances local educational facilities may be employed for the blind child, especially in the earlier years of schooling. The inclusion of handicapped children with normal children is called *mainstreaming*, a popular educational concept at this time.

The child with low vision

In general, children with low vision have great ability to use their residual vision, and they do much better at near than might be anticipated. Children usually have 10 D or more of accommodation and, therefore, have little aversion to holding things close. The use of optical aids by children is ordinarily restricted to those aids that provide significant help. It should be emphasized that near-vision aids are *monocular*. The demands of convergence are greater than can be managed when work is held very near, for example, 10 cm or so. Once the need for a low-vision aid has been established, as with an adult, the trial-and-error method of determining which aid is better is the most successful. Either a high spectacle add or a magnifying glass, hand-held, on a stand, or resting on the page is the most useful. Occasionally, large print books or a television projection device may be used, but this is primarily an educational decision. Some children may benefit from a hand-held telescope for occasional use in seeing distant objects.

Head posture

Head posturing may result in improved visual acuity. Patients with null point nystagmus assume a head posture that places their eyes in the field of vision that reduces or eliminates nystagmus. For example, a patient who has increased nystagmus in right gaze turns his head to the right and maintains his eyes in levoversion in order to achieve a quiet position of the eyes and improved visual acuity. Such patients may go from visual acuity of 20/200 or less in the primary position or in the field of action of their greater nystagmus to 20/40 or better with their head turned in the direction of the greater nystagmus and their eyes turned in their quieter field. Patients with null point nystagmus may hold their head nearly straight for casual seeing and gradually assume a head posture as visual requirements become more demanding. The patients may sit in the examining chair with no head turn and eyes forward, but with pendular or jerk nystagmus. This straight-ahead posture may persist while they read the 20/200 line or the 20/100 line, and gradually as they read more difficult lines the head assumes a posture with the eyes at their null point. Null point nystagmus most commonly is horizontal; that is, the patient turns his head to the right and his eyes to the left in order to assume a quiet field, or vice versa. However, there are instances where null point may be in upgaze, downgaze, or in an oblique field.

The principle of treatment for null point nystagmus is to simulate the neurogenic input of a version while the head remains straight. There are two basic ways to do this. Prisms may be placed with their base toward the direction of head turn. This means that the eyes will be chronically deviated in the direction of the apex of the prism, and a patient who had quiet eyes in eyes right with prisms base-out OS and base-in OD would theoretically have a straight head posture, facing the target, but with eyes in dextroversion and with the nystagmus quieter and visual acuity improved. To an observer, however, the patient appears to be looking to the side rather than straight ahead. Another, more effective method of treating null point nystagmus is the Kestenbaum-Anderson procedure, in which bilateral recession/resections are done to shift the eyes in the direction of the anomalous head turn, so that in order to hold the eyes in the straight, primary position, the eye muscles will require the same neurogenic stimulus as they did preoperatively in lateroversion. Null point nystagmus surgery is effective in the short term, but most studies have indicated that gradually the head posture returns. It has been our experience that surgery offers enough success to warrant it in cases where the head posture causes a cosmetic difficulty to the patient. We have not had patient acceptance of the use of prisms for this purpose.

Null point nystagmus

It is of interest to note that patients with fusion before null point nystagmus surgery have maintained their fusion postoperatively. Some cases of null point nystagmus are complicated by strabismus. These cases require special adjustments to the amount of recession/resection. For head turns in the neighborhood of 30°, we use the 5, 6, 7, 8 "straight flush" type of eye muscle surgery. If a patient has a right head turn and maintains his eyes to the left, our procedure would be left lateral rectus recession of 6 mm, left medial rectus resection 7 mm, right medial rectus recession 5 mm, and right lateral rectus resection 8 mm. The presence of null point nystagmus does not, in our experience, indicate the need for extensive neurologic workup. This is a benign condition that, although persistent, does not indicate other more significant neurologic disease.

Latent nystagmus

Latent nystagmus is relatively common in the pediatric population. It appears in nearly every patient with dissociated vertical deviation and occurs in many patients without. Latent nystagmus may occur with smaller amplitude manifest nystagmus or with perfectly quiet eyes under binocular conditions. Patients with latent nystagmus typically have good vision under binocular conditions but lose one or more lines of acuity when one eye is occluded and the other eye's vision is checked separately. This is a frequent cause of failure of school vision examinations in a patient who otherwise seems to be doing well visually. When such a patient is encountered, his vision should always be checked with both eyes open, and it should be assumed that this is the acuity that the patient uses from a functional standpoint. If it is important to determine the visual acuity of each eye separately, a high plus lens of 6 to 8 diopters can be placed before the untested eye, and acuity can be measured in the other eye without inducing latent nystagmus. Such patients should have a note on their school record indicating that visual acuity checks should be carried out in the binocular state. Latent nystagmus itself, though usually an accompaniment of other types of strabismus, is not a neurologically significant condition.

Hysterical denial of vision

A rare but frustrating type of patient is one who has hysterical denial of vision. This patient is usually a girl in the early to mid teens. The typical behavior is for the child to have a somewhat inappropriate response to an apparent sudden loss of good vision. Worried parents often take the child to several ophthalmologists and are often referred for special evaluations. A common response on vision testing is for such a patient to give an "answer" each time it is asked for on the vision chart. Mistakes are made on the 20/100 line, and the patient continues down to the 20/30 line giving halting answers that are all in error. This should immediately tip off the examiner that the child is actually malingering. With organic or functional vision loss, the cutoff from seeing to nonseeing is more defined. Our practice is to assume a kind but firm attitude and urge the child to respond accurately. In cases where the eye examination has indicated no significant pathologic condition, this technique is usually successful. Often the parents are asked to leave during the examination. We *never* confront this patient, and we urge the family to look for other signs of emotional difficulty while remaining supportive. Management of denial of vision in this manner has been completely successful and, to our knowledge, no repeat "attacks" have occurred.

Special testing methods

A special testing method is the *pinhole test,* the principle of which is that if a small enough pinhole is used (in the neighborhood of 1.5 mm), the light rays that pass through the pinhole and into the eye are parallel to the visual axis, pass through the nodal point, and do not require refraction. Therefore, these light rays are in focus or nearly in focus on the retina without regard for refraction. Testing with the pinhole can result in improved visual acuity in patients with refractive errors or corneal opacities. The pinhole is a quick method for determining if visual acuity is correctable with lenses. In a pediatric ophthalmology practice, younger children may be uncooperative for this test. A brief retinoscopy, placing the proper lens in front of the eyes, may be a quicker test than the pinhole test.

The *random dot stereogram,* as described by Julesz and promoted by Reinecke, may be used as a screening method for visual acuity. Precalibrated random dot figures with directional value can be used to determine minimal visual acuity levels in children but have not received widespread usage.

The *Stycar method,* using the HOTV symbols, in which the patient matches the symbols placed on the screen with symbols that he has in front of him, has been advocated as a useful test, but does not seem to offer any significant advantages over the usual Snellen letters.

Tests to differentiate organic from functional amblyopia

If vision is reduced in one eye and there is a question of whether this reduction in vision has a functional or an organic basis, a simple test can be done to differentiate these two possible causes of decreased vision. The patient is asked to respond to the visual acuity chart using the eye that has reduced acuity while neutral density filters of increasing density are placed in front of the eye. If visual acuity decreases as the density of the filter increases, then organic amblyopia is the cause. If visual acuity remains the same or reduces to a lesser extent than the normal eye as filters of increasing density are placed before the amblyopic eye, functional amblyopia may be diagnosed.

Another method for differentiating organic from functional amblyopia employs the crowding phenomenon. Functionally amblyopic patients demonstrate better visual acuity when responding to single optotypes compared with full-line acuity. Acuity may improve three lines or even more. On the other hand, patients with organic amblyopia have similar acuity levels on both full-line testing and isolated letter testing.

Bead matching may be used in retarded children or very young children in order to get some idea of their minimal separable visual angle.

Forced choice preference test

A newer test called the forced choice preference test is designed to check visual acuity in infants. The child is held by one person, observed by a second, while the third examiner remains behind the viewing board. The examiner, while peeking through a small aperture, observes the patient's preference for formed or unformed objects on the opposite side of the board. The separation of the visual stimuli (stripes) then gives some indication of the visual acuity. This test is time-consuming and has not been used extensively enough to evaluate its ultimate usefulness.

Refraction in pediatric ophthalmology

The refractionist in pediatric ophthalmology must rely heavily on the retinoscope and loose lenses. Small, restless children are not suited for the Phoroptor or automated refractor. In most instances, the objective findings are sufficiently accurate to use to prescribe glasses. In some instances, subjective refraction may be carried out in children, and some pediatric ophthalmologists do this routinely. However, we rarely do subjective refraction on children under 5 years of age. In children 5 and over, a Phoroptor or automated refractor may be useful, but we do not use these instruments. Plus and minus lens bars are useful for very young infants and in the operating room.

In the clinic, the use of loose lenses is greatly facilitated by the practice of "good housekeeping." All lenses should be kept in their holders unless being used for the patient. Our practice is to leave all the tabs in their resting position so that when the final refraction lens has been determined, the tab may be left up, signaling it as the proper lens. When the retinoscopy is concluded, the lenses may then be taken directly from the trial case (with subtraction for the working distance) and placed in a trial frame to check vision. This technique saves a great deal of time and provides more efficiency for the refractionist. Occasionally, a 0.25- or 0.50-diopter Jackson cross cylinder may be helpful in refining the axis and the power of the cylinder in a cooperative patient over 6 or 7 years of age. Either an adult-size or a child-size trial frame is useful in refining refraction in children.

To induce cycloplegia in children under 1 year of age, we use one drop of ½% cyclopentolate (Cyclogyl) and one drop of 2½% phenylephrine (Neo-Synephrine) in each eye and repeat in 1 to 5 minutes. In children over 1 year of age, we use one drop of 1% cyclopentolate and one drop of 10% phenylephrine. In each case, the refraction is done 30 to 40 minutes after the drops have been given. In heavily pigmented children, it may be necessary to double the dosage of dilating drops. In children under 5 with refractive accommodative esotropia, we use ½% atropine solution given 3 days before the refraction. A very specific set of instructions is given to the parents. Stapled to this list of instructions is a ½-cc vial of ½% atropine solution. The parents are instructed to put the drops in the child's right eye in the morning and in the left eye in the evening for the 3 days before the examination, and to put one drop in each eye on the morning of the examination. They are instructed to occlude the puncta when the drops are given and to observe the patient for excess redness or fever. In the event that they have any questions, they are instructed to contact the prescribing ophthalmologist with their questions. After a baseline cycloplegic refraction has been established with ½% atropine, repeat refractions may be carried out using cyclopentolate ½% or 1% or tropicamide (Mydriacyl) ½% or 1%. We do not have 2% cyclopentolate in our clinic.

The refracting instrument of choice is the portable Copeland Streak Retinoscope with a rechargeable battery. This instrument, along with loose lenses, offers a great amount of latitude for the pediatric ophthalmologist, who must remain mobile in order to meet the needs of the patients.

PRESCRIPTION OF GLASSES

When are glasses prescribed? In general, equal, hyperopic refractive errors in patients with straight eyes need no prescription if the refractive error is under 3 to 4 D. If more than 4 D of hyperopia is present, the patient may develop a refractive-type esotropia and also may develop a bilateral, ametropic amblyopia. For this reason, these patients should be watched carefully, and glasses should be prescribed if any indication of strabismus or reduced acuity develops. If the child is examined after 1 year of age, glasses may be prescribed, depending on the family history and on the examiner's assessment of the likelihood of strabismus or amblyopia. As a child gets closer to school age, myopic errors may require correction on an individual basis. In general, the less correction prescribed the better.

Anisometropia plays a special role, since very small degrees of anisometropia can be amblyopiagenic. For this reason, it is necessary to equalize the visual stimuli to each retina as early as possible. It has been our practice to correct over 1 D sph of anisometropia or 1½ D cyl for most children.

Bifocals are prescribed in children for three general situations: (1) nonrefractive accommodative esotropia where the use of a bifocal allows fusion at near, (2) in severely decreased visual acuity where the addition of a high plus bifocal lens allows function at near, and (3) aphakia. The use of low-vision aids in childhood are, in general, limited to the use of high plus bifocal adds. The use of telescopes and hand-held or bar-reading magnifying lenses has limited application. This is not to say that the use of reading aids should not be considered in childhood. They should be used only when it can be clearly demonstrated that the child will both use the device and benefit from it. Bifocals prescribed for motility reasons should have a very high, flat top segment that bisects the pupil. Bifocals for reading purposes should also be large, because in children who require such an add, distance visual acuity will probably not be compromised significantly by the high portion of the add. Parents should be encouraged to get sturdy "sensible" glasses frames for their children. The frames should provide a high glass area. Glass safety lenses are preferred rather than plastic lenses, which are highly susceptible to scratching. The blur appearing in the central aspect of scratched plastic lenses can be troublesome to the patient and may cause significant reduction in visual acuity. On the other hand, scratches in glass lenses tend to be more sparse and, therefore, visually insignificant.

Cosmetic contact lenses are possible in children as young as 5 or 6 years of age, but are not recommended before the mid teens. The important criterion for use of cosmetic contact lenses is motivation on the part of the patient. Children are usually not motivated for contact lens wear before ages 13 to 15. Special indications for contact lenses include correction for unilateral aphakia and the occasional use of pinhole lenses in aniridia (see pp. 150-151). The choice between hard and soft contact lenses is strictly related to the patient; however, in most pediatric applications, hard contact lenses are superior. These lenses are much less expensive, more durable, easier to insert and remove, and easier to clean.

Chapter 2

STRABISMUS

The diagnosis and treatment of patients with strabismus make up a large part of the practice of pediatric ophthalmology. Actually, the subspecialty of pediatric ophthalmology had its origins in the practice of strabismology. This combination of strabismology (which is a disease-related or "vertical" subspecialty) with pediatric ophthalmology (which is an age-related or "horizontal" subspecialty) has produced significant changes in the philosophy of diagnosis and treatment of strabismus as practiced by some. The most important of these changes has been a trend toward earlier intervention. The pediatric ophthalmologist, who is more accustomed to dealing with infants and children, may also be more comfortable with diagnosis and treatment of ocular disease in this young age group. The pediatric ophthalmologist naturally gravitates toward earlier diagnosis, and he will treat children surgically when he thinks the patient will benefit. The most apparent changes in attitude manifested by the pediatric ophthalmologist occur in the treatment of amblyopia and in *early* surgical treatment, especially of *congenital esotropia.*

Several factors must be taken into consideration with regard to strabismus management in the infant and child. What is early surgery? When should the child be first evaluated? How should he be evaluated? When should treatment begin? What should the treatment be? Since no universally agreed-upon definition of early surgery exists, any definition must be considered arbitrary. In general, early surgery is defined as surgery done before the patient is 1 year of age. We have operated on a congenitally esotropic child at 5 months of age, but in most cases by the time the esotropic condition is recognized (by the parents, other relatives, or the pediatrician), referred to the ophthalmologist, adequately worked up, and scheduled, the child is between the ages of 8 and 12 months. The appropriate timing for early surgery varies according to the type of strabismus and the specific needs of the patient. For example, surgery for congenital esotropia is done much earlier in most cases than surgery for intermittent exotropia. Surgery for treatment of vertical muscle anomalies, such as Brown syndrome, congenital superior oblique palsy, double elevator palsy, and congenital third nerve palsy, is done at a later time than congenital esotropia surgery but perhaps earlier than intermittent exotropia surgery.

WORKUP

An argument against early surgery and in favor of deferring surgery until a child is older (2 to 4 years of age or more) is that an adequate workup with adequate measurements cannot be accomplished in an infant. Although this is true in part, experience has shown that precise, objective measurements and reliable subjective responses are not absolute requirements for the successful treatment of congenital esotropia. In other words, it is unnecessary to defer surgery solely on the basis of concern over the precision of measurements. The workup of the infant strabismus patient should, nevertheless, be complete and include the following examinations and procedures.

History

The age of onset and any variations in the strabismus should be noted. The child's birth weight, current weight, and milestones of development should be established to determine the presence or absence of neurologic integrity. Any family history of strabismus or other related diseases should be established.

Visual acuity

A careful visual acuity examination should be done in the manner appropriate for the age of the child (see Chapter 1).

Motility

Testing for *versions*, with special emphasis on determination of cross fixation, and *ductions*, including both having the patient follow an interesting object and testing with the passive doll's head, should be carried out. The angle of deviation may be either estimated by locating the light reflex (Hirshberg's method) or neutralized with a prism held before the fixating eye to center the light reflex in the nonfixating eye (the Krimsky test). In some cases it may be possible to perform the alternate cover test. When the light reflex interpretation is done, an estimated 15 prism diopters ($\triangle$) of strabismus is present for each millimeter of corneal light reflex displacement. When one performs this test, monocular fixation should be examined to determine whether a positive or negative angle kappa exists. When the above tests are used, the deviation in the primary position and in the diagnostic fields of gaze can be estimated fairly accurately. Also, overactions or underactions of muscles can be diagnosed. In the older child, a more accurate measure of the strabismus can be obtained and the presence or absence of dissociated vertical deviation can be determined with the cover-uncover test. (We have not made this diagnosis in patients under 1 year of age.) It is important to recognize that examination should be carried out with the greatest degree of care and accuracy that can be accomplished for a given age patient. However, in our opinion, a worthwhile trade-off can be established between a good estimate coupled with early intervention as compared with a more precise measurement done at a later time with later surgical intervention.

Refraction

Refraction is carried out on all *preschool* children with use of ½% atropine. The dosage is one drop in each eye for 3 days before the examination instilled by the parents at home. For example, a drop is placed in the right eye in the morning and in the left eye in the evening. The puncta are occluded with the parent's finger for a few seconds after the drops are placed in order to cut down systemic effects of the drug. Then a drop is placed in each eye on the day of the examination, for a total of four drops in each eye. This routine provides adequate cycloplegia and does not cause bothersome visual disability to the preschooler. In certain cases where a return office visit for an atropine refraction would impose a hardship on the family, cyclopentolate (Cyclogyl) may be used. For children under 1 year we use cyclopentolate ½%, two drops in each eye, and phenylephrine (Neo-Synephrine) 2½%, two drops in each eye. In children over 1 year of age the dosages are increased to cyclopentolate 1% and phenylephrine 10%. After 30 to 40 minutes, refraction is carried out in young children objectively using the retinoscope and loose lenses.

Fundus examination

Each retina is examined with both the direct and the indirect ophthalmoscope. Most attention is paid to the appearance of the macula and the optic nerve. Study with high plus lenses in the direct ophthalmoscope can also be useful in demonstrating clarity of the media.

Anterior segment

Slit-lamp examination may then be carried out to better assess the cornea, anterior chamber, and lens, but in very young patients the media may be viewed adequately with the ophthalmoscope or by using the retinoscope for retroillumination.

General rules of treatment

As a general rule, patients who, in addition to having strabismus, also have significant refractive error, amblyopia, strabismus with variable deviations, intermittent deviations, or vertical deviation are treated nonsurgically as needed, with a period of observation before definitive surgical treatment is carried out. Patients who have a stable angle, low refractive error, and horizontal deviation (especially an esodeviation) and patients with equal vision and alternation are treated earlier with surgery.

INFANTILE (CONGENITAL) ESOTROPIA (PLATE 2-1)

Infantile esotropia is the most commonly encountered of all strabismus entities. It can be defined as an esodeviation with an onset from birth to 4 months. About 40% of all strabismus patients have infantile esotropia. These patients have moderate to large angles, averaging between 40^Δ and 60^Δ. Because of the techniques of measurement of congenital esotropia, experts often disagree in their measurements, and evidence is lacking that these measurements are significant anyway. If one uses the Hirshberg method of corneal light reflex observation or the Krimsky prism centering of the corneal light reflex, discrepancies of up to 20^Δ can occur. We have seen instances where experienced examiners have disagreed by 20^Δ or more; that is, one examiner estimated that a patient had 40^Δ of esotropia, whereas another equally experienced examiner estimated that the deviation was more than 60^Δ. This can lead to obvious confusion when attempts are made to estimate the amount of correction in prism diopters produced by specific types of surgical intervention. In addition, many of these deviations are highly variable.

When a congenitally esotropic patient is diagnosed and the refractive error is +2.00 D or less and no amblyopia is present, our choice of treatment is early surgery. The surgical treatment of choice is a bimedial rectus recession employing the augmented technique, which consists of recession of the medial rectus muscle measured from the limbus, combined with recession of conjunctiva and Tenon's capsule to the original point of the insertion of the recessed medial rectus muscle. Some patients with infantile esotropia have

34

characteristics of abduction nystagmus and quiet eyes with convergence. They have been called nystagmus blockage or compensation syndrome and have been treated with medial rectus recession and posterior fixation suture. We do not alter our technique of augmented medial rectus recession for these patients. The augmented recession of the medial rectus muscles is carried out in the following manner.

Children under 1 year of age

1. For a deviation of 20^Δ to 25^Δ, the medial rectus muscles are recessed to a point 8.5 mm from the limbus, and the conjunctiva is recessed.
2. For a deviation of 25^Δ to 35^Δ the medial rectus muscles are reattached 9.5 mm from the limbus, and the conjunctiva is recessed.
3. For deviations of 35^Δ to 50^Δ or more, the medial rectus muscles are reattached at 10.5 mm from the limbus, and the conjunctiva is recessed.

PLATE 2-1

Characteristics of congenital esotropia.
Onset: Birth to 4 months.
Angle: 50^Δ (average).
Refractive error: +1.50 D (average).
Amblyopia: Infrequent.
Treatment: (1) If amblyopia is present, *occlusion* until alternation; (2) if no amblyopia is present or after alternation is achieved, *surgery,* augmented recession as early as possible.

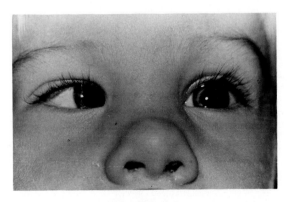

PLATE 2-1

PLATE 2-2

Augmented recession of the medial rectus muscles.

A A limbal incision extending from the 1 o'clock to the 5 o'clock meridian in the right eye and the 11 o'clock to the 7 o'clock meridian in the left eye.

B After the muscle is freed of its intermuscular attachments, secured with suture, and dissected from the globe, the reattachment point is measured from the limbus according to the schedule noted.

C The muscle is reattached to the sclera with 5-0 or 6-0 synthetic absorbable suture.

D The conjunctiva is closed at the muscle's original insertion with 8-0 synthetic absorbable suture.

E **(1** and **2)** Preoperative 70$^\Delta$ congenital esotropia; **(3)** postoperative straight with minimal conjunctival scar.

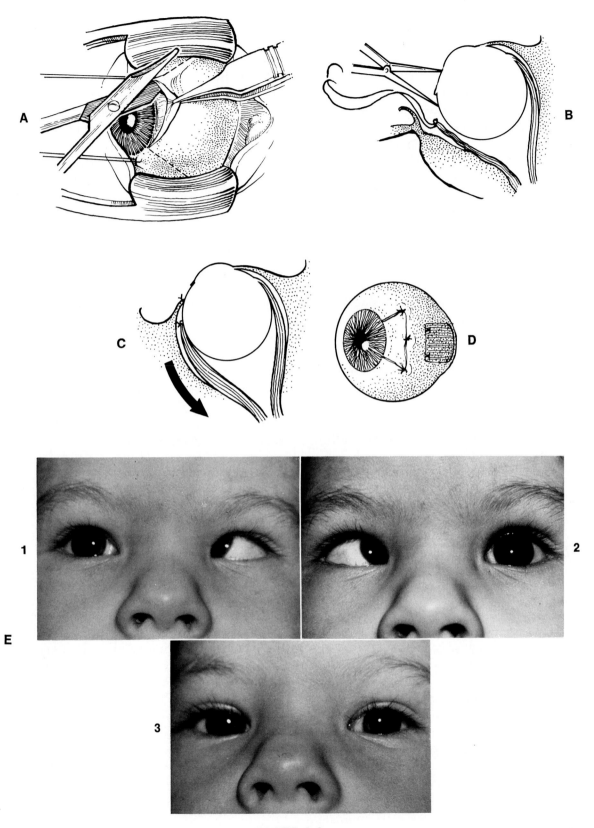

PLATE 2-2

37

Children over 1 year of age

Because the globe is larger in older children, 0.5 mm is added to each medial rectus recession measurement. In essence, congenital esotropia is measured as small, medium, and large; and bimedial rectus, en bloc recessions are graded as small, medium, and large. The surgeon may titrate for deviations between, and he may vary from these figures if he is not obtaining a fairly equal number of overcorrections and undercorrections. This formula, in our hands, places three out of four patients within 10^Δ of straight in the early (6 months postoperative) course.

Dissociated vertical deviation

Seventy-five percent of surgically treated congenitally esotropic patients should be corrected to within 10^Δ of being straight, 10% require early reoperation for overcorrection or undercorrection, and 15% have more than 10^Δ of residual strabismus but are cosmetically acceptable. Anywhere from 50% to 90% of successfully treated congenital esotropic patients develop dissociated vertical deviation (DVD) from 6 months to 3 years or more after successful esotropia surgery. Of these patients, approximately 10% will require surgery for cosmetically objectionable DVD. Our surgical procedure of choice for DVD is a superior rectus recession and posterior fixation suture on one or both eyes. If one eye is habitually used for fixation and only the nonpreferred eye manifests a hyperdeviation, this eye alone is done. For DVD of 10^Δ, a 3.5-mm superior rectus recession is combined with a posterior fixation suture attaching the superior belly of the superior rectus muscle to the sclera at a point 12 mm posterior to the superior rectus muscle's original insertion. If the vertical deviation is 30^Δ, the superior rectus muscle is recessed 5 to 6 mm with the posterior fixation suture placed 12 mm from the original insertion. Persistent DVD is treated with a second procedure, which is an inferior rectus resection of 3.5 to 6.0 mm. A very large DVD of greater than 30^Δ may be treated with a large superior rectus recession and posterior fixation suture plus an inferior rectus resection of 5 mm. In cases where free alternation exists and either eye may be hyperdeviated from DVD, superior rectus recession with a posterior fixation suture may be done bilaterally.

What are the benefits derived from early surgery for congenital esotropia? We are not aware of any study that provides convincing evidence that early surgery produces a definite improvement in function compared with later surgery. On the other hand, we are unaware of any clear-cut evidence that significant benefit is gained by waiting until a child is older before performing surgery for congenital esotropia. Our philosophy has been that if the child derives no benefit other than straighter eyes at an earlier age, early surgery for congenital esotropia is justified. In addition, it seems logical that for a given child, the earlier the eyes are straight or nearly straight, the better will be the chance for development of binocular vision with at least peripheral fusion. Therefore, since no compelling reason exists for deferring surgery, we elect to do surgery as early as the appropriate workup and (if necessary) treatment of amblyopia can be completed.

ANESTHETIC RISKS OF EARLY SURGERY

It has been common for ophthalmologists to express concern that general anesthesia is unsafe for very young children, particularly those under 1 year of age. More specifically, the argument is presented that if one is unable to show clear-cut benefits from early surgery, the added risk of anesthesia to the infant is not worth taking. This assumption that there is an added risk is not valid, provided competent pediatric anesthesiologists are available (see Chapter 13).

CHILDHOOD EXODEVIATIONS
Infantile and childhood exotropia

Childhood exotropia is much less common than esotropia. However, infantile exotropia does exist. We have seen several children who have demonstrated frank exotropia from the first few weeks of life. This type of exotropia usually disappears. However, if exotropia has been diagnosed and is present past 6 months of age, and if other contraindicating factors, such as amblyopia, muscle palsies, mechanical restrictions, and cerebral palsy, have been excluded, surgery may be done. We have operated on exotropic patients before 1 year of age, but rarely. In such a case, an appropriate-size recession of the lateral rectus muscle and resection of the medial rectus muscle should be carried out.

Childhood intermittent exotropia

Intermittent exotropia in childhood is considered a "safe" strabismus. It usually is noticed for the first time when the child is between 1 and 3 years old. The parents note that the child is not looking at them properly. They may even say that one eye goes "in." In this case they are referring to the recovery movement rather than the manifest deviation. When called upon to examine an intermittent exotropic child, we carry out the usual strabismus diagnostic routine. Our treatment program, however, is more restrained than with congenital esotropia. After the initial examination, the family is sent home with a type of "report card." The family is asked to make note of the following: How often is the eye out? How long does the eye remain out? How readily is the refusion process carried out? Is the deviation getting "better" or "worse"? Does the child close one eye when outside in bright sunlight? Early in the evaluation the parents should be shown the extent of the exodeviation and the character of the refixation movement. Cover testing should be carried out while the child fixates on far distant objects, at least 200 feet away. If a child maintains a fairly steady pattern of intermittent exotropia, has good vision in each eye, and maintains fusion with good stereopsis at near, he may be followed safely for months to years. On the other hand, if there is any deterioration in the fusion ability with increasing periods of manifest deviation and decreasing periods of fusion with decreasing quality of fusion, surgery should be carried out earlier. There are significant differences of opinion regarding philosophy of treatment for intermittent exotropia. Many highly qualified pediatric ophthalmologists and strabismus surgeons urge early surgery for intermittent exotropia as they do for congenital esotropia, and others urge the use of overminus spectacles to control the exodeviation.

PLATE 2-3

Infantile and childhood exodeviations.

A Six-month-old infant with exotropia.

B Intermittent exotropia in an 8-month-old child.

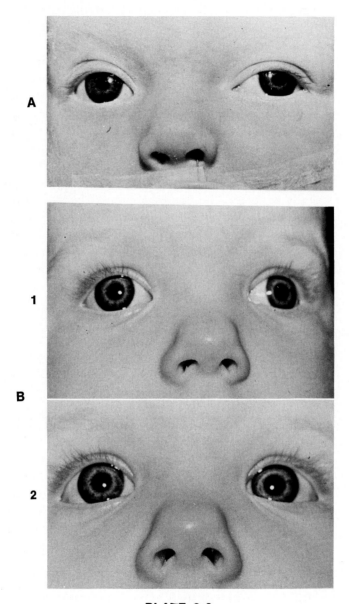

A

1

B

2

PLATE 2-3

REFRACTIVE AND NONREFRACTIVE ACCOMMODATIVE ESODEVIATIONS
Refractive accommodative esotropia

Refractive esotropia is an esodeviation that occurs as a natural result of a normal accommodation convergence/accommodation (AC/A) ratio in uncorrected hyperopia. Refractive esotropia usually occurs between ages 2 and 3 in a patient who has a moderate to high hyperopia in the range of +4.00 D or more. The esodeviation begins when the patient becomes more interested in looking at objects close at hand. An uncorrected hyperopic refractive error in this range in the presence of adequate accommodative ability puts a great strain on the fusional divergence mechanism. When fusional divergence is overcome, the eyes become esodeviated. Such a patient with uncorrected hyperopia has the "choice" of seeing a single blurred image or a doubled image in which one is clear and one is blurred. In a very short time, the second blurred image is suppressed, and either alternation or amblyopia supervenes. The timely prescription and use of spectacles with repeat refractions and careful follow-up provide adequate treatment for refractive esotropia in most cases. If glasses are not provided soon enough or if the hyperopia is not fully corrected, the esodeviation may become refractory to optical treatment and require surgery. If glasses are worn faithfully and strong fusional patterns are established (especially if the hyperopia decreases), many refractive esotropia patients can manage straight eyes without wearing glasses by the time the teen years are reached. The use of anticholinesterase drops or ointment in such patients with a normal AC/A ratio is not an adequate substitute for glasses.

Nonrefractive accommodative esotropia

The patient with accommodative esotropia is unique in that a high AC/A ratio is combined with low hyperopia or even myopia. These patients have either straight eyes or a moderate esotropia in the distance with a much larger esotropia at near. Amblyopia is frequently present if the condition remains untreated. As with refractive accommodative esotropia, nonrefractive accommodative esotropia ordinarily becomes evident between ages 2 and 3 years. The treatment consists of full correction for the distance refractive error with the addition of bifocals for near. Our choice of bifocal treatment is to give these patients +3.00 lenses with a flat top, high segment bifocal that *bisects the pupil*. This does not mean the spectacle lenses are bisected, because in most instances there is more glass below the center of the pupil than above. It is very important that bifocal glasses be fitted properly in these children. The management of accommodative esotropia can be difficult and frustrating because these people may be extremely variable in their ability to fuse in spite of faithful wearing of their glasses. DFP ointment or echothiophate (Phospholine Iodide) drops 0.125% or 0.06% given as often as every day in each eye or as infrequently as is required may be used to help these children maintain bifoveal fusion at near. Careful, regular follow-up, repeat refractions, and amblyopia treatment are required in all these patients. These patients are followed for many years, but fortunately most of them can be weaned of their bifocals by the early teen years or even younger. There are two basic philos-

PLATE 2-4

A Refractive accommodative esotropia **(1)** with and **(2)** without +4.00-D correction.

B A properly placed bifocal should have the segment top bisect the pupil in the primary position. **(1)** Distance fixation through carrier; **(2)** near fixation through carrier; **(3)** near fixation through add.

C A properly written prescription for bifocals for nonrefractive accommodative esotropia includes explicit instructions for the optician with a sketch included.

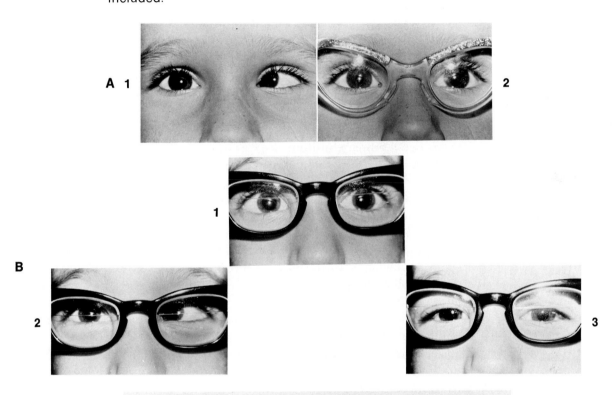

PLATE 2-4

ophies for weaning from bifocals. Some ophthalmologists prefer to reduce the strength of the bifocal in 0.5- to 1-D increments as the fusion at near becomes better maintained. Other ophthalmologists prefer to retain the full +3.00 add until the patient is able to fuse at near without bifocals altogether, limiting near tasks or using the glasses intermittently when necessary.

OTHER TYPES OF CHILDHOOD STRABISMUS
Duane syndrome

Duane syndrome may occur with the eyes esotropic, exotropic, or straight in the primary position. This strabismus is characterized by narrowing of the palpebral fissure and enophthalmos on attempted adduction. Also, an upshoot or, less commonly, a downshoot of the affected eye occurs during adduction. Duane syndrome may be unilateral or bilateral, but usually affects the left eye in women, and is commonly associated with Goldenhar syndrome (hemifacial microsomia). Duane syndrome is treated surgically if one of the following conditions exist: (1) a cosmetically objectionable head posture that is assumed to obtain fusion, (2) a cosmetically objectionable strabismus, usually an eso-tropia in the primary position, or (3) a cosmetically objectionable narrowing of the fissure with enophthalmos on attempted adduction.

The treatment scheme differs for each manifestation of Duane syndrome. If the esodeviation in the primary position is the reason for surgery, a reces-sion of the medial rectus muscle on the involved side is carried out. If the eyes are relatively straight but an enophthalmos is the biggest problem, both the medial and lateral rectus muscles of the involved eye may be recessed. If some esodeviation in the primary position exists, the muscles may be re-cessed different amounts so that a straightening in the primary position is effected. If exotropia is present, the lateral rectus muscle is recessed. In pa-tients in whom no significant enophthalmos or lid retraction is present, a full tendon transfer shifting the superior and inferior rectus muscles to a point adjacent to the lateral rectus muscle may be carried out. There may be some question as to whether these patients really have Duane syndrome or whether congenital sixth nerve palsy is present. In patients in whom the esodeviation is severe and the lid retraction and enophthalmos are also severe, a three-re-cession procedure may be carried out. This includes a recession of the medial and lateral rectus muscles on the involved eye and recession of the medial rectus muscle on the uninvolved eye. Surgery for Duane syndrome should be deferred in most instances until the child is approaching or in the school years.

PLATE 2-5

A Duane syndrome OS. **(1)** Eyes are straight in the primary position; **(2)** the fissure of the left eye narrows as the eye becomes enophthalmic on at-tempted adduction; **(3)** abduction of the left eye is possible only a few de-grees beyond the midline.

B **(1)** Duane syndrome with a slight esotropia OS; **(2)** the left eye upshoots on attempted adduction; and **(3)** the fissure widens as the left eye attempts to abduct.

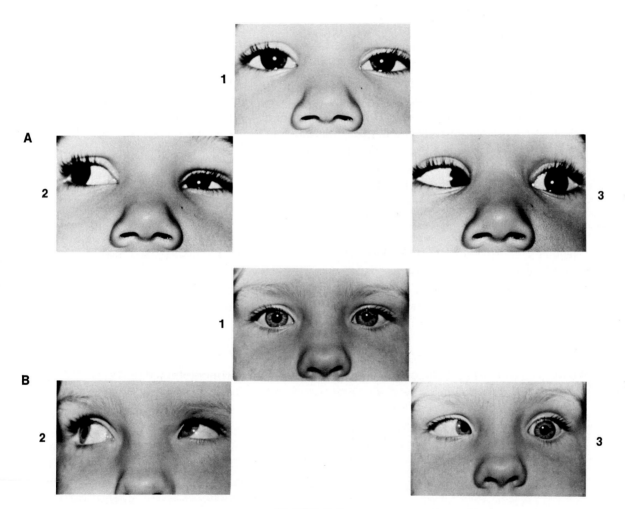

PLATE 2-5

Congenital superior oblique palsy

Congenital superior oblique palsy is not unusual; it occurs in approximately 25% of all patients who have superior oblique palsy. Superior oblique palsy is usually evident by the time the child begins to walk. The first manifestation of congenital superior oblique palsy is often an abnormal head posture. This consists of a head tilt to the opposite side with depression of the chin. This condition must be differentiated from the orthopedically caused torticollis. Differentiation seems to be more difficult from the orthopedic view than from the ophthalmologic view. Superior oblique palsy may be treated surgically when the patient is 3 to 5 years old. Of note, congenital superior oblique palsy has not usually, in our experience, produced a torsional response when patients are tested with the double Maddox rod, whereas patients with acquired unilateral superior oblique palsy exhibit a response when tested with the double Maddox rod, indicating an excyclotorsion averaging 7° to 8°.

The treatment scheme for superior oblique palsy consists of weakening the antagonist, strengthening the agonist, or weakening the yoke muscle. We have not seen cases of bilateral congenital superior oblique palsy. However, we have seen one case of bilaterally absent superior oblique muscles occurring in a patient with a bizarre incomitant exotropia with V pattern and four cases where one superior oblique muscle was absent congenitally. The Knapp classification scheme for surgical treatment of superior oblique palsy is useful.

Some cases of adult superior oblique palsy that have no apparent cause are in all likelihood decompensated cases of congenital superior oblique palsy. These patients have enormous vertical fusional vergence amplitudes, which are sufficient to control their deviation in childhood but eventually prove to be inadequate between the third and fifth decade.

PLATE 2-6

A The head posture assumed as a result of congenital left superior oblique palsy in a 7-year-old boy. The head is tilted to the right, and the chin is depressed. This head posture allows the eyes to be used in a field away from that of the paretic left superior oblique muscle.

B **(1)** In the primary position, a small left hypertropia is present; **(2)** a larger left hypertropia is present in dextroversion, and **(3)** the eyes are straight in levoversion. **(4)** the left hypertropia is greater on head tilt to the left compared with **(5)** head tilt to the right. This indicates a left superior oblique palsy in this 4-year-old girl.

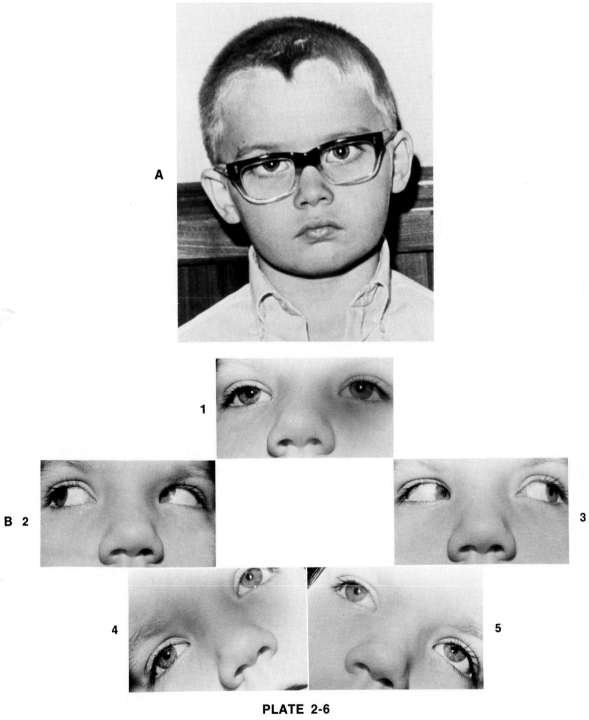

PLATE 2-6

Brown superior oblique tendon syndrome

Brown syndrome occurs for a variety of reasons, but always results in a relative inability of one or both eyes to elevate fully in adduction. Brown syndrome should be treated surgically only if the head posture is objectionable or if a hypodeviation or secondary hyperdeviation causes a cosmetic strabismus problem. Surgery should be done when the patient is in the toddler to preschool years and consists in most cases of a superior oblique tenotomy or recession. The important part of treatment of Brown syndrome is finding and then freeing the restriction to elevation in adduction. The surgical treatment of Brown syndrome is one of the least predictable surgical procedures of the extraocular muscles, primarily because of the varied and multiple etiologies of the syndrome.

PLATE 2-7

A Brown syndrome is present when the trochlear — superior oblique insertion distance cannot increase because of mechanical causes. *(1)* This may be due to inability of the superior oblique tendon to pass freely through the trochlea, *(2)* a fibrous band along the reflected superior oblique tendon, *(3)* a tight tuck (iatrogenic), or *(4)* restrictions elsewhere.

B **(1)** The eyes are straight in the primary position, but **(2)** the right eye fails to elevate in adduction. Brown syndrome is confirmed by finding resistance to passive elevation of the right eye.

C Acquired, traumatic Brown syndrome of the left eye caused by a German shepherd bite.

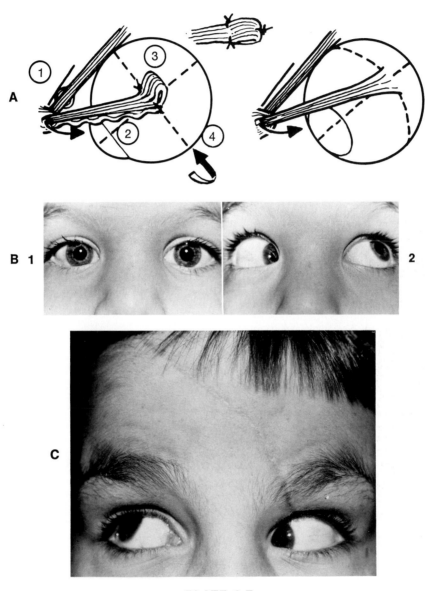

PLATE 2-7

Double elevator palsy

Double elevator palsy occurs with or without ptosis and with or without mechanical restriction to elevation, but invariably demonstrates a hypodeviation of the involved eye. It is treated when the patient is in the toddler to preschool years by freeing the restriction of the antagonist muscle when necessary and doing either a full tendon or rectus muscle union transfer to the superior rectus muscle.

PLATE 2-8

A Left hypotropia and ptosis in the primary position in a patient with congenital double elevator palsy.

B On attempted upgaze, the left eye demonstrates limited elevation.

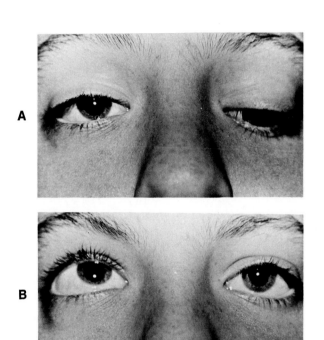

PLATE 2-8

Double depressor palsy

Double depressor palsy is much less common than double elevator palsy. Double depressor palsy is treated by freeing any mechanical restrictions to depression and then doing a full tendon transfer or rectus muscle union transfer to the inferior rectus muscle. Most cases of significant limitation to depression are acquired from trauma involving the inferior rectus muscle with mechanical entrapment, denervation, or both.

Congenital third nerve palsy

The patient with congenital third nerve palsy has large exotropia, small hypotropia, and ptosis. The pupil may also be dilated. This condition may be bilateral or unilateral and may occur in an otherwise normal child or more commonly in a child who has cerebral palsy or mild to severe mental retardation. The treatment of choice for congenital third nerve palsy is a large lateral rectus recession combined with a superior oblique tendon transfer. The superior oblique tendon is removed from the trochlea and is shortened and reattached to the sclera at the point just above the insertion of the medial rectus muscle. During the same procedure a frontalis suspension of the upper lid may be carried out. This surgery may be done when the patient is between 1 and 2 years old.

PLATE 2-9

A Bilateral congenital third nerve palsy in a 2-year-old boy.
B When the child is asked to look upward while the lids are elevated by the examiner, no elevation or adduction of either eye takes place.
C The same patient at age 5 years, 3 years after undergoing a bilateral lateral rectus recession of 8 mm and a bilateral superior oblique tendon transfer, in which the cut end of the reflected superior oblique tendon was attached to the sclera just superior to the insertion of the medial rectus muscle.

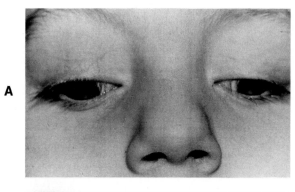

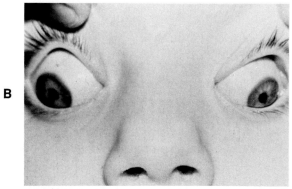

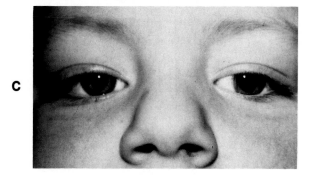

PLATE 2-9

Congenital sixth nerve palsy

Congenital sixth nerve palsy must be differentiated from Duane syndrome and congenital esotropia. In congenital sixth nerve palsy, the mechanical restriction to passive abduction is less or may be absent. If some restriction to abduction is present, it is due to secondary contracture of the antagonist medial rectus muscle. The Jensen muscle tendon union with recession of the medial rectus muscle is carried out when there is significantly restricted passive abduction; a full tendon transfer is carried out when there is no significant restriction to abduction.

Infantile sixth nerve palsy

Infantile sixth nerve palsy may occur after a viral illness or as a result of trauma or increased intracranial pressure from any cause. All the usual factors in following any type of sixth nerve palsy should be considered. However, careful patching of infants and children to avoid amblyopia and suppression should be carried out while one waits for the lateral rectus muscle to recover.

Möbius syndrome

Möbius syndrome is an esotropia caused by a congenital sixth and seventh nerve palsy. The patients have moderate to large angle esotropia, inability to abduct either eye, flattened nasolabial folds, atrophy of the distal third of the tongue, and a history of poor feeding. Möbius syndrome is treated surgically with a large bimedial rectus recession and conjunctival recession with or without bilateral lateral rectus resections. Surgery is done before the patient is of school age.

Simultaneous contraction of the lateral rectus muscles

Simultaneous contraction of the lateral rectus muscles (perversion of the extraocular muscles) is an extremely rare congenital strabismus that has been reported in only a handful of cases. In this condition, Hering's law is broken. When the eyes attempt a lateral version, both lateral rectus muscles contract in one or both gaze positions. The one case of this type we observed occurred in a 2-year-old boy with arthrogryposis multiplex congenita. His father was Caucasian and his mother Oriental.

PLATE 2-10

A This patient demonstrates the typical findings of Möbius syndrome. In spite of a rather dull appearance, these patients have normal intelligence. Children with Möbius syndrome tend to look alike.

B **(1)** In the primary position this boy with simultaneous contraction of the lateral rectus muscles has 90$^\Delta$ of exotropia; **(2)** on attempted levoversion, the right eye *abducts,* increasing the exodeviation; **(3)** on attempted dextroversion, a convergence-like response occurs, and the exodeviation decreases somewhat.

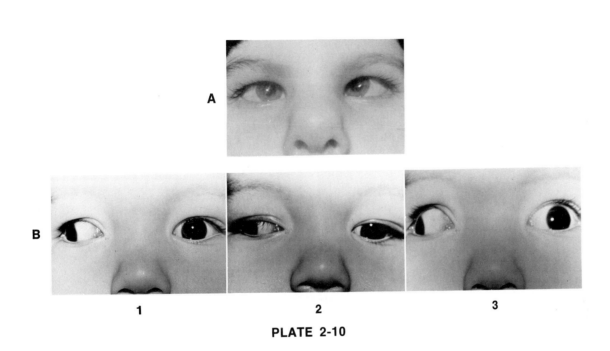

A

B

1   2   3

PLATE 2-10

Fibrosis syndrome

Fibrosis syndrome is characterized by a hypodeviation of both eyes and bilateral ptosis with reduced or absent levator function. On attempted elevation the eyes become spastically esotropic. This condition is transmitted as an autosomal dominant trait. It should be treated with an inferior rectus recession and a bimedial rectus recession with bilateral frontalis suspension of the upper lid. Surgery should be carried out when the patient is in the toddler years.

PLATE 2-11

A This patient with fibrosis syndrome has eyes that are hypodeviated and slightly esodeviated while he looks approximately in the primary position.
B On downgaze the eyes become moderately exodeviated.
C When upgaze is attempted, a spasm of convergence occurs with a marked increase in the esodeviation.

Oculomotor apraxia

Oculomotor apraxia is a rare condition in which the supranuclear connection for voluntary movements of the eyes is absent or deficient. The eyes are repositioned by the labyrinthine system for pursuit movements. To do this, the head is rotated in the direction the eyes are to be moved until the eyes take up fixation. The head then rotates back until the eyes are centered in the palpebral fissure and maintain fixation. This condition is nonthreatening to the patient, and no treatment is available. Reading is always difficult for these patients.

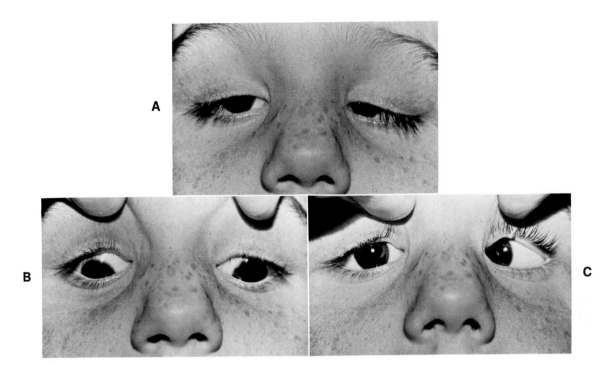

PLATE 2-11

Chapter 3

AMBLYOPIA

Amblyopia has been defined by von Noorden[32] as "a unilateral or bilateral decrease of visual acuity caused by form deprivation, abnormal binocular interaction, or both, for which no organic cause can be detected by physical examination of the eye and which, in appropriate cases, is reversible by therapeutic means." An extraneural organic cause of decreased visual acuity, such as cataract, astigmatism, strabismus, or an uncorrected bilateral or unilateral refractive error, serves as a trigger mechanism that produces a functional visual decrease in a susceptible individual. This decreased vision on the basis of inadequate visual input usually persists after the amblyopiagenic factor, such as the cataract or refractive error, has been removed and after the usual mechanisms of remediation, including optical therapy, have been accomplished in an otherwise normal eye. Active antisuppression treatment (usually in the form of occlusion of the preferred eye) must be carried out, in addition to elimination of the amblyopiagenic factor in the young patient to reverse the amblyopia. Strabismic amblyopia can be treated successfully by patching, with or without straightening the eye.

The incidence of amblyopia is in the neighborhood of 2% of the population and, therefore, is of real socioeconomic importance. The presence of amblyopia may reduce the involved individual's effectiveness in the job market and certainly increases the potential impact of injury to the better eye.

The extent of visual loss in amblyopia varies. Minimal loss of as little as one line 20/25 OD, 20/20 OS could be on a functional basis and be reversible, although not disabling. On the other hand, functional amblyopia may cause visual acuity loss to 20/200, 20/400, or even worse, which, if persisting in older childhood or adulthood, may be difficult or impossible to reverse. For statistical purposes and in most studies, two lines or more of reduction in visual acuity in an otherwise normal eye are required for the diagnosis of amblyopia.

CLASSIFICATION
Strabismic amblyopia

Strabismic amblyopia occurs in an individual with strabismus who habitually suppresses the same eye on a subconscious level to avoid diplopia. Cross fixation (that is, using the left eye for right gaze and the right eye for left gaze) and free alternation are the antitheses of strabismic amblyopia, and when these conditions occur, amblyopia does not exist.

Anisometropic amblyopia

Anisometropic amblyopia occurs when an uncorrected difference in refractive error between the two eyes produces one retinal image that is relatively out of focus compared with the other. The more blurred image (usually from the more ametropic eye) will be suppressed. This type of amblyopia may lead to a small-angle manifest strabismus or may persist with no apparent strabismus, in which case microtropia or monofixational syndrome exists.

Deprivation amblyopia

Deprivation amblyopia occurs in one or both eyes when the eye receives a deficient input of light and form, or no input at all. Unilateral or bilateral cataracts are the most common causes of deprivation amblyopia. Corneal scarring, ptosis, and bilateral ametropic amblyopia can also lead to deprivation amblyopia.

The association of form deprivation and abnormal binocular interaction as dual and sometimes overlapping and reinforcing mechanisms in amblyopia must be recognized and treated adequately in the management of the patient with amblyopia. Suppression combined with deficient visual input is a potent amblyopiagenic factor. Bilateral visual deprivation from bilateral congenital cataracts and ametropic amblyopia is, in general, more amenable to treatment than amblyopia with a suppression component.

MECHANISMS

PLATE 3-1

A *Strabismic amblyopia* results from abnormal binocular interaction because the fovea of each eye views a different object and transmits this image to the occipital cortex. Only one image is the object of regard, the other being suppressed after confusion and diplopia are overcome. Also, form deprivation occurs, since the deviated eye invariably presents a blurred image because the object seen by the fovea of the deviating eye will be at a different point in space than the object seen by the fixating eye. This image will be out of focus because the deviating eye receives the same accommodative input as the fixating eye.

B *Anisometropic amblyopia* also results from a dual amblyopiagenic mechanism. The fixating eye has a clear image, whereas the anisometropic eye has a blurred image, which causes unequal binocular input and leads to suppression of this eye. In addition, the suppressed eye (usually the more ametropic eye) invariably becomes strabismic either with a microtropia or a small-angle deviation.

60

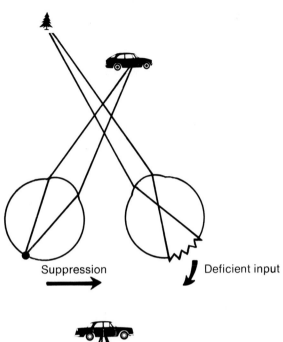

Suppression

Deficient input

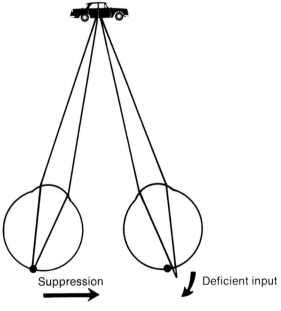

Suppression

Deficient input

PLATE 3-1

61

PLATE 3-2

A Unilateral cataract or unilateral media opacities also produce a dual amblyopiagenic mechanism. The blurred image from the involved eye represents the visual deprivation part, and the suppression of this blurred image by the fixating eye contributes the abnormal interaction aspect.

B Bilateral congenital cataracts or media opacities cause only form deprivation amblyopia.

C Ametropic amblyopia from uncorrected bilateral high hyperopia also causes amblyopia only from form deprivation factors.

Electrophysiologic studies of animal models of amblyopia have shown that decreased cortical firing is produced by the amblyopic eye, regardless of the mechanism for amblyopia.

Anatomic studies of behaviorally confirmed amblyopic primates have shown cellular changes in the lateral geniculate body subserving the amblyopic eye.

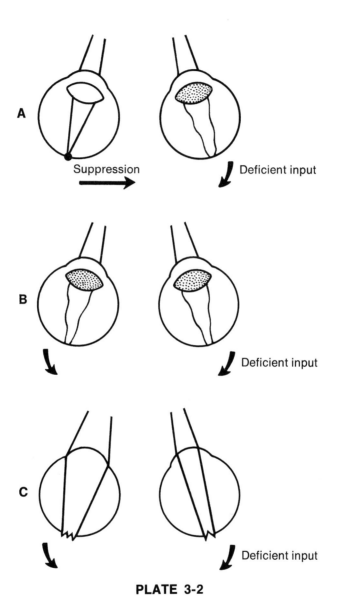

PLATE 3-2

AGE OF SUSCEPTIBILITY AND TREATMENT

The human is at risk to develop functional amblyopia from any of the previously stated causes until age 6 or 7 years. After this time, the onset of strabismus or the occurrence of any other potentially amblyopiagenic factors, such as an acquired cataract, is unlikely to cause amblyopia. In the event of an acquired visual defect after this age, even one that persists for months or years, vision should return to normal or near normal after the cataract or other impairment is removed and appropriate measures have been taken for optical correction.

Just as the years from birth to 6 or 7 years old are the ages of susceptibility for amblyopia, they are also the ages when amblyopia is most successfully treated. In general, the younger the patient, the more rapidly he will develop amblyopia from any cause and the more rapidly he may be treated successfully for amblyopia by appropriate treatment methods, such as patching. If amblyopia remains untreated until after the age of 6 to 9 years, the visual defect may be irreversible. The precise cutoff age for susceptibility and treatability of amblyopia cannot be established with certainty. There may be individual variations; also, the precise age of onset of amblyopia cannot be determined with accuracy in every case. It is a good rule of thumb to say that an individual with any level of functional amblyopia can regain the best level of vision that he has ever had in the visually mature amblyopic eye, provided the proper therapeutic measures are undertaken or provided that he loses visual acuity in the formerly preferred eye to a level below that of the currently amblyopic eye. Because of this, it seems reasonable that an amblyopic eye, regardless of the age of the child, deserves at least one sincere attempt at treatment, regardless of when this treatment is begun. If several weeks or months of patching result in no improvement, then irreversible amblyopia may be said to exist.

DIAGNOSIS

The diagnosis of amblyopia requires both a demonstration of visual acuity loss and the absence of an organic cause. However, in the presence of an extraneural organic cause, such as unilateral or bilateral cataract or anisometropia, amblyopia can still be inferred because we know that in such cases functional amblyopia will persist even after the amblyopiagenic factor has been eliminated.

Visual acuity also can be diagnosed from objective evaluation of the fixation behavior. The more unsteady the fixation and the more preferred the fellow eye, the poorer is the vision in the nonpreferred eye. Eccentric fixation is always associated with decreased vision. This is diagnosed by determining that an area of the retina other than the fovea is used as the principal visual direction. The farther this acquired nonfoveal principal visual direction is from the fovea, the poorer the visual acuity will be. However, in some cases, amblyopia is present in spite of central fixation.

Full-line acuity is the only accurate and reproducible method for determining vision in functional amblyopia. Because of the crowding phenomenon, visual acuity tested with single optotypes may produce erroneously good visual results. Acuity in the amblyopic eye is also relatively better in reduced illumination. The neutral density filter test may be used to differentiate functional amblyopia from organic amblyopia. With filters of increasing density, a normal eye or an eye with an organic visual defect will show gradually reduced visual acuity response. On the other hand, a functionally amblyopic eye will have vision that remains the same or is reduced less when compared with a normal eye.

TREATMENT

The treatment modalities for amblyopia include *occlusion* (complete or incomplete, constant or intermittent), *penalization* (distance, near, or both), and *pleoptics*. The principal treatment for amblyopia is occlusion of the preferred eye. The type of treatment that is most suitable depends on the age of the patient and the type of amblyopia.

The treatment of amblyopia must always begin with the removal or modification of the amblyopiagenic factors when possible. This means glasses should be prescribed for bilateral high hyperopia and for anisometropia of 1 D sph or 1.5 D cyl. Obstructions in the media must be eliminated, and appropriate optical correction provided.

Patching routine
Strabismic amblyopia in children under 1 year

Amblyopia is diagnosed when children demonstrate strong preference for fixation with one eye. These children should have full-time patching (all the waking hours) begun as soon as the diagnosis is made. On the day patching is begun, a 1-week return appointment should be made. Parents should be instructed to observe the infant's fixation pattern at least once each day. If the parents observe that the fixation preference has been shifted from the patched eye to the nonpatched eye, the patch should be shifted to the formerly amblyopic eye and alternate patching should be carried out until the patient returns. When alternation is achieved, surgery is done in most cases of congenital esotropia. Von Noorden suggests that children under 1 year of age should have the preferred eye patched for 3 days and the amblyopic eye patched for 1 day as a beginning routine. The important fact to realize is that severe patch amblyopia can develop in an infant, and that during the patching routine, one eye should always remain patched to avoid recurrence of suppression.

Strabismic amblyopia in children older than 1 year

The preferred eye is patched full-time, and the family is instructed to watch for changes in fixation pattern and for alternation at the time when the patch is off briefly before bedtime. A return appointment is made for 2 weeks, and thereafter at 1-month intervals until alternation is achieved or until there is no improvement in vision noted for a period of 2 to 3 months. If full-time patching has been faithfully applied, after 2 to 3 months of no improvement, consideration should be given to discontinuing the patch. Our policy is to continue patching only if the parents are anxious to continue or if there is some suspicion that patching has not been applied as faithfully as indicated by the family.

Anisometropic amblyopia

Anisometropic amblyopia is usually diagnosed later than other forms of amblyopia because in most cases the eyes are grossly straight and there is no physical manifestation to call attention to this defect. Often, children are picked up in vision screening checks at age 3 or 4 or at preschool vision tests when they are 5. Initial treatment for anisometropic amblyopia is to provide the child with full correction or a reduced spherical correction with the reduction carried out equally in diopters between the eyes. The glasses are worn for 2 to 6 weeks. At this time, visual acuity is rechecked, and if the amblyopia persists, a careful patching program is begun. The preferred eye is patched full-time, but careful observation is carred out to ensure that occlusion strabismus has not developed. It is especially important in occlusion therapy in patients who have amblyopia and straight eyes to make sure that hyperopia is adequately corrected. Uncorrected hyperopia can make the amblyopic patient more prone to develop occlusion strabismus.

Amblyopia after unilateral aphakia

Probably the most difficult amblyopia to treat is that which occurs in cases of unilateral cataracts. These patients suffer from the dual causes of amblyopia: (1) form and light deprivation and (2) abnormal binocular interaction. The onset of the amblyopiagenic factors is from birth or shortly after, and the patients have no chance whatever to develop any type of normal vision in the affected eye. Treatment consists of removal of the cataract followed by prompt, accurate aphakic correction usually with a contact lens and patching of the normal eye. Unfortunately, in spite of the most vigorous effort, these patients seldom obtain vision of better than the 20/200 to 20/100 range. Some claims of visual acuity of 20/40 or even 20/30 are made, but these instances are indeed rare and subject to confirmation. In cases where a contact lens is not tolerated and patching is refused, we have treated patients with spectacles for use for just a few hours a day coupled with patching of the phakic eye. The visual rehabilitation of these unilateral aphakic patients is probably the most discouraging of all amblyopia problems.

Bilateral aphakia

The visual rehabilitation in the patient treated for bilateral cataracts is much more straightforward and successful. Care should be taken to remove the cataracts with the briefest possible interoperative interval in order to avoid the risk of creating the same situation as occurs in the patient treated for unilateral cataract. Bilaterally aphakic patients are usually treated with spectacle correction, although contact lenses and bifocals may be worn by the older child.

Recurring amblyopia

Not infrequently, amblyopia is treated to a point where vision is stabilized with a line or two of decreased vision in the amblyopic eye. In many of these cases, when patching is discontinued, the previously amblyopic eye will slip several lines in visual acuity. When this occurs, patching the good eye just a few hours a day during a period of visual use may reverse the pattern and restore better acuity in the amblyopic eye. This course of part-time, complete occlusion may be carried out for many years even until the child is a teenager. Usually, after this time all enthusiasm for even part-time occlusion is gone. One of the realities of treating a patient with this type of amblyopia should be pointed out: a person who has visual acuity of 20/20 in each eye but who has strabismus with alternation will have visual acuity that could be tested under binocular conditions at less than 20/200 in the nonpreferred eye at any time. Much the same is true in the amblyopic patient who has 20/20 vision in one eye and perhaps 20/40 vision in the other eye but with a small-angle strabismus and no bifoveal fusion. These acuities are tested under monocular conditions and represent *potential* vision. In everyday seeing, in spite of having 20/40 vision potential in the nonpreferred eye, the patient has vision of 20/200 or less under usual binocular seeing conditions. The importance of demonstrating good vision in the amblyopic eye is that this visual acuity could be called upon when needed if vision becomes reduced in the preferred eye. Although binocular acuity is reduced in the nonpreferred amblyopic eye, the visual field afforded by this amblyopic eye is extremely useful, and the amblyopic patient or the patient with strabismus who has a preferred eye is certainly functionally better off than a person with only one seeing eye.

Penalization

Amblyopia may be treated successfully by providing the preferred eye with a blurred image and the amblyopic eye with a cleared image. This is best done by fully atropinizing the preferred eye and withholding hyperopic correction. At the same time, the amblyopic eye is given full distance correction and in some cases a bifocal to enhance near visual acuity. In this instance, penalization is carried out in the preferred eye both for distance and for near. The effectiveness of penalization is enhanced if some hyperopia exists in the preferred eye. If the preferred eye is not hyperopic, a minus lens may be placed in front of this fully atropinized eye to accomplish distance penalization. This also enhances near penalization in the atropinized eye. Other, more complicated schemes have been devised for penalization, but they do not add much to the picture of amblyopia treatment. Penalization seems to work best when acuity has been improved by other means to the 20/80 level or better.

Partial occlusion

On-glass occlusion may be carried out in a variety of ways. An opaque clip may be placed over the lens. Scotch tape in the form of magic mending tape may be used to frost the glass. A cosmetically acceptable, clear-appearing glass that produces a very blurred image may be employed. Bangerter or graded filters may be used, or in some cases a Fresnel prism is used to provide a slight amount of blurring to the preferred eye in instances of minimal amblyopia. All these on-glass occlusion techniques have the same inherent weakness. That is, the patient can rather easily look around this occluder if he wishes to see better. On-glass occlusion has few indications in cooperative or motivated patients. Strip or segmental on-glass occlusion has no place whatever in the treatment of amblyopia. A high plus or opaque contact lens may be used for occlusion of the preferred eye, but the expense and morbidity of a contact lens make this type of treatment usable only in very specific cases. Some ophthalmologists have advocated gluing the eyelashes together on the preferred eye or even sewing the lids together. This extreme treatment is rare if used at all. A black cloth (pirate patch) is preferred by some patients, but these have a habit of slipping, and patients using them are prone to peeking. Twenty-four-hour, on-face occlusion is advocated by some, but this represents a degree of treatment that is probably not any more effective than conscientiously applied waking hour occlusion.

Pleoptics

Designed to reestablish the superiority of the fovea, pleoptics is the technique specifically applied to the treatment of eccentric fixation. Of course, eccentric fixation is always accompanied by amblyopia. In pleoptics the fovea is stimulated either actively by afterimages or passively by parafoveal dazzling. The treatment technique originated in Europe and was popular in the early 1950s. It has recently been determined that pleoptics offers no clear-cut advantage over standard occlusion techniques in the treatment of amblyopia with or without eccentric fixation.

Inverse occlusion or occlusion of the amblyopic eye in order to reduce some of the adaptation that occurs in eccentric fixation is also probably of little value. A red filter placed before the amblyopic eye in cases of eccentric fixation likewise has little established value.

If pleoptics has any value, it is in the adult patient with long-standing amblyopia and eccentric fixation who loses his good eye. Perhaps pleoptics in this instance will hasten the recovery period in the amblyopic eye, but will in all likelihood have no beneficial effect over and above the natural course of visual restoration created by the loss of the good eye.

Phase contrast grating

A claim has been made that brief periods of occlusion combined with near vision tasks done against a background of rotating vertical stripes greatly reduce treatment time for amblyopia. Although it is well known that patching therapy is more effective if the amblyopic eye is used, the value of phase contrast grating has not been established and remains subject to confirmation.

SUMMARY

Amblyopia treatment as well as amblyopia prevention is an important part of pediatric ophthalmology. Vision salvaged through restoration of good acuity in a functionally amblyopic eye represents a worthwhile saving of a human resource.

Chapter 4

CHILDHOOD CATARACTS

Lens opacities are seen frequently in children as well as in adults. Most of these opacities are sutural opacities and do not interfere with vision. The anterior axial embryonal opacity is so common as to be considered a variant of normal. Clinically significant lens opacities from any cause are relatively rare in children, and the term cataract should be used only to describe those lens opacities that interfere with vision. Needless concern and anxiety can be spared parents if the examining physician refers to an insignificant lens opacity by a term other than cataract and uses instead the terms opacity or spot to describe these insignificant findings.

Significant childhood cataracts, on the other hand, are an important cause of visual deprivation because they interrupt the process of visual development and maturation. In studies of the etiologies of blindness in children, congenital cataracts can be shown to comprise from 10% to 38% of the total. Visual results after treatment are better now than in the past, but as will be pointed out later in this chapter, the visual results from cataract surgery for certain types of cataracts remain unsatisfactory. Therefore, cataracts continue to be a significant cause of visual loss in children.

INCIDENCE

The incidence of congenital cataracts is said to be 1 in 250 live births.[9] Sutural lens opacities may be present in as many as 20% or 25% of normal individuals, while other small, discrete opacities may be seen in 90% or more of the population. Congenital cataracts are hereditary in from 8% to 23% of cases. The autosomal dominant form of cataract is most frequently seen, followed by autosomal recessive, and then sex-linked cataracts, which are rather rare. In certain populations in which childhood cataracts occur, trauma is the leading etiologic factor. Congenital idiopathic cataracts and lens opacities related to persistent hyperplastic vitreous also occur frequently. Other developmental anomalies and mental retardation are seen with increased frequency in patients with congenital cataracts. Indeed, most congenital anomalies do not occur in isolation but rather in association with defects in other organ systems.

69

PATIENT ASSESSMENT

The assessment of a young patient with cataracts should begin, of course, with a careful family history. The history may provide a clue to the etiology of the cataract, and further etiologic workup may not be necessary. The most important question to be answered in this initial assessment, however, is whether the cataracts are progressive. It may be difficult to lend credence to the history given by the family in some cases, because the described progression of a cataract may turn out to be erroneous with the family having only recently become aware of a cataract that was, in fact, present from birth. On the other hand, when they do occur, developmental cataracts are the most important of all to recognize and must not be overlooked, because prompt surgery and appropriate aphakic correction may prevent dense amblyopia in a visually immature patient. Depending on the age of the child, mechanical causes may be the most likely cause of cataract, particularly unilateral cataract. Metabolic cataracts may be reversed or their development stopped.

DEVELOPMENTAL CATARACTS
Cataracts of trauma

The older child is more susceptible to injury, and a clear history of trauma usually can be obtained in cases where it exists. On the other hand, young infants, particularly when victims of the battered child syndrome, may have traumatic cataracts without a valid history of trauma.

Cataracts of prematurity

Prematurity is associated with several intraocular abnormalities, including a transient form of myopia and so-called cataracts of prematurity. Remnants of the tunica vasculosa lentis and of the pupillary membrane are commonly found in these infants and account for transient and insignificant opacities of the lens that are readily seen with the direct ophthalmoscope. Although retrolental fibroplasia is cited as a frequent cause of cataracts in this group of infants, our experience has been that when the retinopathy is that severe, the lens opacities are insignificant in comparison. The lens tends to become more cloudy with age, and many children in their second decade who are victims of retrolental fibroplasia develop a progressive cataract. This cataract usually absorbs, partially or completely, and presents as a membranous cataract or a cataract with significant membranous element.

Cataracts due to defective posterior capsule

Another cataract that we have seen with some frequency is developmental and, in our experience, presents as a bilateral, congenital cataract but with a true developmental history. We have been able to make the diagnosis preoperatively in some cases in which the lens opacity did not preclude viewing the posterior capsular area. All cases, however, were definitively diagnosed at the time of surgery. A posterior subcapsular plaque is not an unusual finding in congenital cataracts, but in this group of patients, the posterior plaque incorporating the posterior capsule centrally allows the escape of watery material that is readily seen with the operating microscope at the time of less aspira-

70

tion. Vitreous does not escape, and the anterior hyaloid face remains intact. By increasing the intraocular pressure with the infusion, a funnel-shaped excavation can be seen to extend deep into the vitreous cavity, which seems to be in excess of the depression one could force onto the vitreous face by merely increasing intraocular pressure anterior to it. The clear history of progressive cataracts and the bilateral nature of seven of these cases we have observed personally lead us to speculate that the cataract is indeed developmental and is due to a defective posterior capsule that overlies the area of attachment of the primary vitreous, which fills the funnel-shaped defect in the vitreous. A rent in the defective posterior lens capsule allows ingress of fluid and subsequent cataract development. This condition is to be contrasted with posterior lenticonus, which is usually unilateral and is associated with a double ring reflex on retinoscopy and has the typical biomicroscopic findings of a posteriorly bulging lens capsule.

Galactosemia cataracts

Galactosemia cataracts undoubtedly are among the most important developmental cataracts to recognize and treat. They are said to occur in over 75% of patients with abnormal galactose metabolism, and onset is a few days or a few weeks after birth. The cataract has been described as an "oil droplet" type of cataract in its early development. These cataracts are always progressive if untreated, whereas early treatment halts the cataractous process and reverses intermediate lens changes. The defect in galactose metabolism is due to an enzyme deficiency of either galactose-1-phosphate uridyl transferase or galactokinase. Galactokinase deficiency is less common and has a more benign course with few systemic implications. Cataract may be the only significant finding in galactokinase deficiency, whereas galactose-1-phosphate uridyl transferase deficiency is associated with mental retardation, hepatomegaly, splenomegaly, diarrhea and vomiting, weight loss, and death if untreated.

The diagnosis of these disorders is readily established by demonstration of elevated blood galactose levels and enzyme. Loading doses of galactose can be given to parents or siblings as well as to the patient in selected cases to more readily establish the diagnosis. Red blood cell assays for the suspect enzyme may also be done. The easiest, least expensive screening test, a urinalysis, may reveal albuminuria in addition to reducing substances when tested by Clinitest (rather than testing specifically for glucose).

Zonular cataracts

Zonular cataracts may suggest a diagnosis of tetany or metabolic dysfunction but in fact are usually hereditary. Any young patient being evaluated for cataracts should be examined with the biomicroscope in order to establish the precise anatomic location of the lens abnormalities. Embryonal cataracts are never metabolic and need not be worked up for metabolic reasons. An infant born with a zonular cataract, which encompasses the fetal nucleus and therefore essentially the entire lens at birth, probably has a hereditary form of zonular cataract. On the other hand, if this area of the lens around the fetal nucleus becomes opacified after birth, an exogenous cause for this cataract must be suspected and appropriate laboratory investigation undertaken. Patients

71

with metabolic zonular cataract have a history of one or more episodes of tetany in about half the cases. Dental hypoplasia is present in approximately half the cases, and ricketts is present in about one fourth the cases. A history of hypocalcemia can be uncovered, therefore, in a significant number of patients who have zonular cataracts due to metabolic causes. Other metabolic cataracts do occur in children, however. Diabetes mellitus has been reported as causing the cataracts of a 1-year-old child. The typical snowflake appearance of diabetic cataract is not often seen in children under 10 years of age, being more common in teenagers and young adults. The hypoglycemic, hyperkalemic cataract described by Wilson[46] and others probably occurs more often than recognized and is a true metabolic cataract. Hypothyroidism is not a common cause of cataracts in children but remains a consideration in undiagnosed cases. Myotonic dystrophy is suspect as a metabolic cause but does cause irridescent lens opacities in young people and has been reported in children younger than 10 years of age.

Cataracts due to infection, inflammation, or medication

Cataracts of infectious or inflammatory etiology can be suspected by noting associated intraocular inflammatory findings such as synechiae or by associated systemic findings such as juvenile rheumatoid arthritis. The most common cataract of this type is the rubella cataract, which is often unilateral and may or may not be associated with glaucoma. Cataracts occur commonly as a consequence of intraocular infection, although the presence of trauma in many of these cases makes it difficult to ascertain what is due to the trauma and what is due to the subsequent infection.

Cataracts associated with juvenile rheumatoid arthritis have been particularly troublesome because of the associated intraocular inflammation, the significant presence of band-shaped keratopathy, and the slow but progressively downhill nature of this disorder.

Steroids are often used in these patients, although the beneficial effect on ocular inflammation has been questioned. The disease process as well as the medication causes cataracts. Usually these cataracts have a significant posterior subcapsular component. Our experience has been that we have not seen cataracts caused by steroids in a child when it could be ascertained that the steroid and not the inflammatory process was the causative agent. Phospholine iodide has been implicated as a cause of cataracts, but only one case of transient anterior subcapsular vacuoles has been reported in children, and it seems that this drug is safe if used with discretion and if stopped when lens changes appear.

Cataracts due to dermatologic disorders

Cataracts associated with dermatologic disorders include those cataracts with an anterior capsular component. The presence of ichthyosis, Rothmund-Thomson syndrome, Werner syndrome, atopic dermatitis, poikiloderma, or a similar skin disorder should alert the clinician to the possible association with the cataract. Any chronic skin disorder in a patient with cataracts should be investigated as a possible explanation for the presence of the cataract.

Cataracts due to inborn errors of metabolism

Several inborn errors of metabolism have been associated with cataracts.

Alport syndrome, which consists of hereditary nephritis, deafness, and cataract, is usually diagnosed by family history, the presence of urinary abnormalities, and associated signs and symptoms.

Fabry disease, angiokeratoma corporis diffusum, is a peculiar disorder characterized by a whorllike corneal dystrophy, posterior spokelike cataracts, and angiokeratoma in the bathing trunk area. This is a disorder of sphingolipid metabolism and is a storage disease. The enzyme, ceramide trihexosidase, is deficient.

Lowe syndrome consists of mental retardation, congenital cataract, and glaucoma. This is an sex-linked, recessive disorder, although similar findings have been reported in females. Aminoaciduria is present.

Homocystinuria, hyperlysinemia, and sulfite oxidase deficiency are known to be associated with lens subluxation, but it appears that most of the disorders that cause subluxated lenses also produce a cataract, probably due to the mechanics of the subluxation itself.

Wilson disease, a disorder of copper metabolism, is well known for the Kayser-Fleischer ring seen on the cornea, but so-called sunflower cataract, primarily an anterior capsular cataract, is also pathognomonic of the disorder. The trisomy syndromes (trisomy 13, trisomy 16 and 18, and trisomy 21) have a high incidence of cataracts. Other congenital disorders in which cataracts occur frequently are of the syndromes of Conradi, Hallermann-Streiff, incontinentia pigmenti, and any of the syndromes associated with retinitis pigmentosa, such as Laurence-Moon-Biedl.

DIAGNOSTIC EVALUATION

Diagnostic evaluation, therefore, of any patient with congenital or early onset cataracts should begin with taking a careful history. This will obviate significant or unusual investigative studies in the majority of cases. An ophthalmic evaluation, including a biomicroscopic examination to localize precisely the cataract to the portion of the lens most involved and to ascertain the presence or absence of intraocular inflammation, is mandatory.

Even the smallest infant can be examined with the slit lamp, if patience is employed and ancillary help is used. An examination with the patient anesthetized is rarely necessary, although this is indicated if the examination cannot be accomplished in the usual clinical setting. The physical examination should determine the presence or absence of associated systemic abnormalities. A minimum workup of a patient with congenital cataract should include a urinalysis, with emphasis on testing for reducing substances in general rather than glucose specifically, serum calcium and phosphorus, a genetic urine screen for metabolic disease, and enzyme studies as appropriate. It has been suggested that all patients with developmental cataracts be taken off milk immediately, with the resumption of milk feeding only after a diagnosis other than galactosemia has been established. This seems to be easily accomplished and is a reasonable suggestion.

Additional studies that can be obtained in questionable cases include blood urea nitrogen or creatinine for renal disease, FTA-ABS for syphilis, rubella titers, urine tests with ferric chloride for phenylketonuria, or urine sodium nitroprusside or serum methionine levels for homocystinuria. Serum copper will be low in Wilson disease, but the most reliable test for Wilson disease is a 24-hour urine copper quantitative determination, which will be high if the patient has the disorder.

TREATMENT OF CHILDHOOD CATARACTS

Any clinically significant lens opacity (cataract) in childhood should receive prompt attention because of the possibility that deprivation or suppression amblyopia will develop. This type of amblyopia is more likely to occur in younger children up to 6 or 7 years of age. Unilateral cataracts are more amblyopiagenic than bilateral. When bilateral, complete cataracts are more amblyopiagenic than incomplete cataracts, although visual results have not yet provided any firm justification for this. On theoretical grounds, unilateral cataracts should be treated as early as possible if surgery is to be done at all. Surgery on unilateral congenital cataracts has been reported as early as the first few days of life, but timing of surgery has to be done with the knowledge of the infant's general health and with the family's ability to cooperate in the infant's care.

Other treatment options for childhood cataract include chronic dilatation or optical iridectomy. Optical iridectomy has not been employed by us and probably has few indications in the treatment of childhood cataracts.

Lens removal should be followed by prompt aphakic correction, employing a contact lens or spectacles with an add for near. In virtually all instances, occlusion therapy of the noninvolved eye will be required.

Surgical options

Extracapsular cataract extraction is the most widely employed technique for treatment of congenital and acquired cataracts in children. Modern techniques for extracapsular lens removal combine constant anterior chamber infusion with needle aspiration of the lens material. The constant irrigation produced by infusion, combined with aspiration that occurs essentially at the same rate, allows the soft eye of the infant to retain its shape during the surgical procedure, reduces the likelihood of extensive vitreous loss, and prevents unnecessary traction on the vitreous base and retina. Irrigation may be supplied through a needle placed in a second corneal incision separate from the irrigation instrument. Aspiration may be carried out with or without the aid of a variety of cutting, emulsifying, or fragmenting instruments, but since most cataracts in children are soft and aspirate readily with a moderate amount of suction, no special instrument is required in most cases.

In some instances, hard, calciumlike plaques or segments require additional time for aspiration, but most of these can be removed also without great difficulty, using simple aspiration. However, the lens capsule itself and secondary membranes that may form after a prior aspiration or after injury to the lens cannot be aspirated and must be incised with scissors or a knife or chopped and aspirated with a sharp, reciprocating cutting instrument and aspiration.

74

Decision making

PLATE 4-1

A A small, hard white punctate lesion may be seen located in the center of one or both lenses. The opacity may be slightly anterior or slightly posterior. This insignificant cataract requires no treatment. This type of cataract is not progressive.

B Sutural opacities appear as featherlike changes on the lens' suture lines and therefore, appear in roughly a Y-shaped pattern. These cataracts are usually bilateral but asymmetrical. In most cases, these cataracts are an insignificant finding and require no treatment.

C Segmental cataracts are usually unilateral and often appear to be associated with developmental defects of a colobomatous type. These cataracts are rarely progressive, but if they do progress, the cataract may require removal.

D Zonular cataracts are usually bilateral and roughly equal in density. This cataract may have occurred as a result of neonatal tetany or because of some transient prenatal or postnatal event that went undiagnosed. Often these cataracts are inherited. These opacities are best been in retroillumination. They may be mild and occasionally may be noted on a routine examination and may not cause any significant decrease in vision. When a child reaches the age where visual acuity can be determined, such cataracts may reduce visual acuity a line or two. If visual acuity is good in these eyes, nothing need be done about the cataracts. These cataracts may be progressive or may be dense enough to reduce visual acuity. If so, removal of the cataract in one or both eyes is indicated.

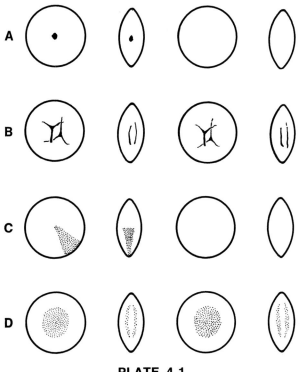

PLATE 4-1

75

PLATE 4-2

A Zonular cataracts with cortical rider opacities are usually bilateral and are of varying density. These cataracts must be judged on their own merit with regard to vision. If visual acuity is decreased significantly, one or both cataracts should be removed.

B Posterior capsular and subcapsular cataracts may be seen in very young children, in whom they are often congenital and unilateral, or they may represent metabolic or complicated cataract in an older child, in which case the cataracts are bilateral. These cataracts are usually dense, centrally located, and create a severe impairment to vision. When congenital and unilateral, the postoperative management is difficult, and a full understanding on the part of the physician and the parents must be present before treatment is undertaken. Bilateral acquired posterior capsular cataracts have a much better prognosis for useful vision.

C Anterior polar cataracts are usually unilateral and densely white. A projection is frequently seen coming forward from the anterior lens capsule. These cataracts are removed for functional reasons if large but are not significant most of the time. Older children or young adults may have an amblyopic eye but with a dense opacity in the pupil that is objectionable because of its appearance. Consideration may be given for removal in this instance.

D We have seen a bilateral posterior capsular progressive cataract in seven patients. The posterior capsule at the border of the opacity may rupture, and fluid that fills the funnel-shaped defect in the vitreous comes forward into the lens and causes total opacity of the lens. At the time of removal of these cataracts, the funnel-shaped defect may be enlarged or allowed to collapse without vitreous loss. We feel that this is a peculiar type of developmental cataract related to anomalous vitreous formation. These cataracts are similar to those seen in posterior lenticonus, but in typical posterior lenticonus the vitreous anomaly is not seen.

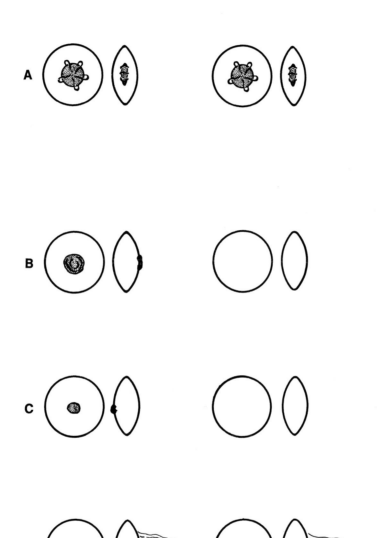

PLATE 4-2

PLATE 4-3

A A blue dot, or cerulean, cataract is usually bilateral, and although it decreases visual acuity somewhat, it is not clinically significant nor does it often require removal. Some of these patients may have a progressive increase in density in their cataracts, but this is usually slow.

B Persistent hyperplastic primary vitreous (PHPV) is usually unilateral and causes a dense posterior capsular cataract of variable size associated with a persistent hyaloid stalk. This stalk – posterior capsule union may tear the lens capsule, causing sudden maturity of the cataract. These lenses may be removed, but vision is seldom restored. Removal may be indicated to reduce traction on the ciliary body, thereby improving the integrity of the eye.

C Unilateral complete or mature cataracts may occur as a primary event or as a progression of an incomplete cataract such as that which occurs suddenly when a PHPV plaque ruptures the posterior capsule. These cataracts should be removed.

D Bilateral, complete, or nearly complete congenital cataracts should be treated with early surgery. It is important to note that there should be a minimum interval between surgery on the two eyes. This is to reduce the likelihood of anisometropic amblyopia.

The treatment of bilateral cataract is made simpler by the fact that surgical decisions are easier. The surgical timing of bilateral cataract surgery is not as restrictive as with unilateral cataracts. Unilateral cataracts are more amblyopiagenic than bilateral cataracts, but on the other hand, undue delay need not occur in the treatment of bilateral cataracts.

In the young child, a decision as to cataract surgery must be made on the basis of the ophthalmologist's experience and judgment of the degree of visual impairment the lens opacities are producing. Visual behavior will be important, but the decision for or against surgery must be made without visual acuity numbers. In general, if a clear reason for cataract removal does not exist, it is better to wait until the child is older, when a numerical acuity, accurate assessment of visual capabilities, progress in school, and other factors can be determined.

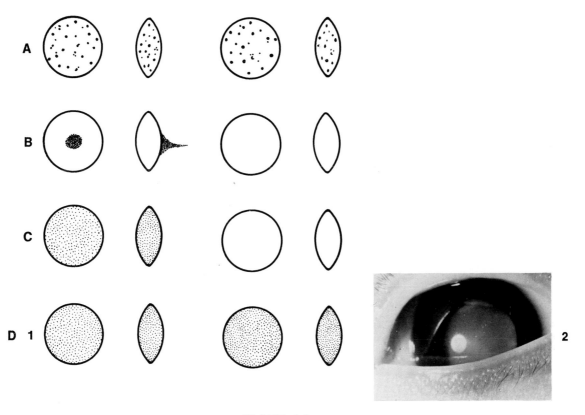

A

B

C

D 1

2

PLATE 4-3

CATARACTS AND ANTERIOR SEGMENT TRAUMA

PLATE 4-4

A Cataracts after severe eye trauma should be treated in the acute period with one stage surgery in most instances. The corneal or corneoscleral laceration is repaired, any iris prolapse is excised or replaced in the anterior chamber, and as a second stage of this procedure, discission and aspiration of the lens material is carried out.

B A secondary membrane with Elschnig pearls after an extracapsular cataract extraction is indication for surgical treatment. The Elschnig pearls and lens material may be aspirated, but the posterior capsule, if present, must be either incised or, if it is fibrotic and thickened, chopped and aspirated with an instrument such as the Ocutome.

C An old, partially resorbed traumatic cataract with anterior and posterior synechiae is treated by lysis of the synechiae, followed by revision of the pupil and cutting and aspiration of the lens contents and capsule.

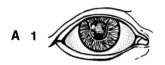 A 1 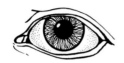 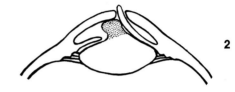 2

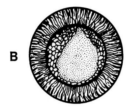 B

C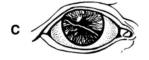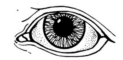

PLATE 4-4

81

INFANTILE CATARACTS

Clinical evaluation of an infantile cataract can be much more difficult than the same procedure done in an adult. Children will not cooperate readily for subjective examination, of course, and objective examinations with the slit lamp are difficult. A useful scheme for evaluation of infantile cataracts can be carried out in five steps, the last four of which are illustrated in Plate 4-5.

First, some estimation of visual acuity is obtained by objective means. Children with dense unilateral cataracts object severely to occlusion of one eye. In cases like this, they actually push the examiner's hand away. Children with significant bilateral cataracts manifest decreased awareness of their surroundings and often have a wandering pendular type of nystagmus. Of course, older children who can cooperate for visual acuity testing should have vision determined in this manner.

When these tests are completed, the decision whether to remove the cataract can be made. Unfortunately, matters are not clear-cut at this point. For example, when discussing the possibilities of cataract surgery with the family of a 3-month-old child with a dense unilateral cataract, the surgeon must be honest in stating that the probability of obtaining visual acuity of better than 20/200 or 20/100 in spite of the most vigorous optical correction is poor. On the other hand, if any hope at all of obtaining useful vision is to be entertained, the cataract should be removed. Parents are given as many reasons for not doing the cataract surgery as for doing it. It is not proper to create guilt feelings in parents who decide not to have the surgery done, but on the other hand, it is unfair to withhold the opportunity to have the cataract removed. Some families feel that they are derelict in their duty if they do not have the cataract removed. They consider the cataract as a blemish and attach other significance to its presence. For whatever reason, if, after a careful explanation with an honest representation of both sides, the family wants to have the cataract removed, plans should be made for early surgery. Of course, the rigors of postoperative visual care are explained to the family in great detail. In the case of a unilateral cataract, this includes the use of a contact lens on the operated eye and a patch on the good eye for several hours a day. In cases where contact lens treatment is a total failure, spectacles are prescribed.

PLATE 4-5

A Objective evaluation of lens clarity is carried out with the ophthalmoscope on a high plus lens power setting. Lens material usually appears white or bright, and the configuration of the cataract itself can be seen. This examination provides only indirect information with regard to how well the patient can see.

B The retinoscope can be employed for retroillumination. With the retinoscope light focused on the retina, the cataract appears as a black shadow. This assessment provides a good estimate of how much occlusion to the visual axis the cataract is producing.

C Retina examination with the direct and the indirect ophthalmoscope also provides some information as to how effectively the light passes through the media to the retina.

D The patient should be examined with the biomicroscope. This can be done in almost every instance, although in very young children it requires one or two people to support the child's chin on the instrument. In cases in which the retina cannot be seen, ultrasound examination with the A or B scan, or both, should be done to provide information about the integrity of the retina and the vitreous space.

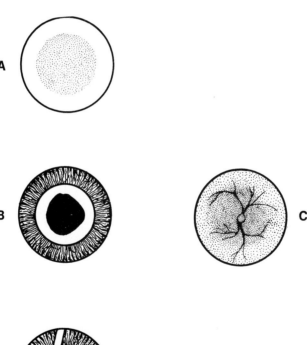

PLATE 4-5

SURGICAL TECHNIQUE
Discission and aspiration

All infantile cataract operations are performed with the operating microscope. The pupils are dilated widely preoperatively, using 0.5% or 1% cyclopentolate and phenylephrine 10%. After being anesthetized using endotracheal anesthesia, the patient is positioned with his or her head at the end of the table in a secure head rest.

PLATE 4-6

A A solid blade blepharostat is used to separate the lids, and a 4-0 or 5-0 black silk suture is placed in the insertion of the superior rectus muscle for traction. This suture is then secured with a serrefine or small hemostat. Some surgeons prefer to place a stabilizing or traction suture in the inferior rectus muscle also.

B For surgery on the right eye, a shelving incision is made in clear cornea, at the 7 o'clock position, using a No. 75 Beaver blade. This incision is enlarged to approximately 1 mm with a serrated McCaslin knife.

C A 3-inch length of No. 50 polyethylene tube that has been placed over a 23-gauge butterfly scalp vein needle is inserted into the anterior chamber. The scalp vein needle is connected to a 1-liter bottle of lactated Ringer solution, which is 1 meter above the level of the patient's head. At this time, care should be taken to see that the intraocular pressure is not elevated excessively.

D The same No. 75 Beaver blade is used to enter the anterior chamber through clear cornea, at the 12 o'clock position. At this time, irrigation fluid will run out of this incision, and intraocular pressure will only be mildly elevated.

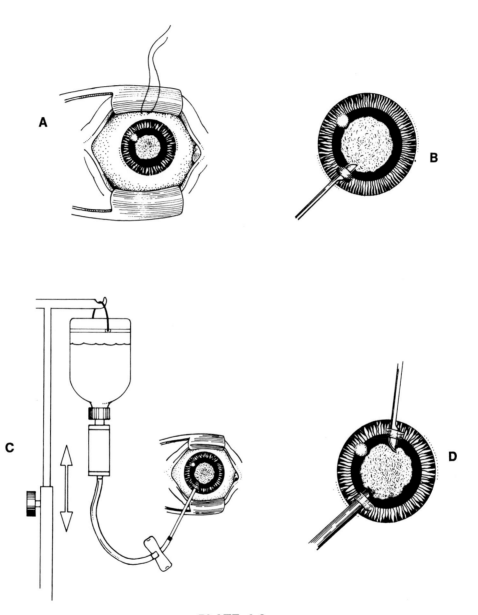

PLATE 4-6

PLATE 4-7

A The anterior capsule may be opened in a variety of ways. **(1)** A cruciate incision may be made or multiple linear incisions in the anterior capsule may be made or **(2)** the anterior capsule may be removed in a can-opener fashion. Our choice is to use a disposable 27-gauge needle that is bent on its tip to form a type of cutting hook. This is placed on a 2-cc syringe and is inserted into the anterior chamber through the superior incision. Multiple, small, equatorial incisions are made in the anterior capsule of the lens. The capsule is peeled toward the 12 o'clock incision. **(3)** The capsule is brought up through the incision and excised with small scissors. **(4)** If it is impossible to bring the capsule out through the incision with the 27-gauge needle, a fine forceps is used to grasp the capsule and withdraw it from the superior incision, where it is excised as completely as possible.

B A 22-gauge, end-aspirating Gass needle is then placed into the anterior chamber and gently thrust into the substance of the lens material at the six o'clock position. A gentle but firm backward pull is placed on the plunger and the lens material is aspirated into the syringe. In some cases an entire lens can be aspirated without removing the syringe. In other cases multiple removals and reapplication of the syringe may be required. Removal of the lens material requires a certain feel on the part of the surgeon, which must be experienced.

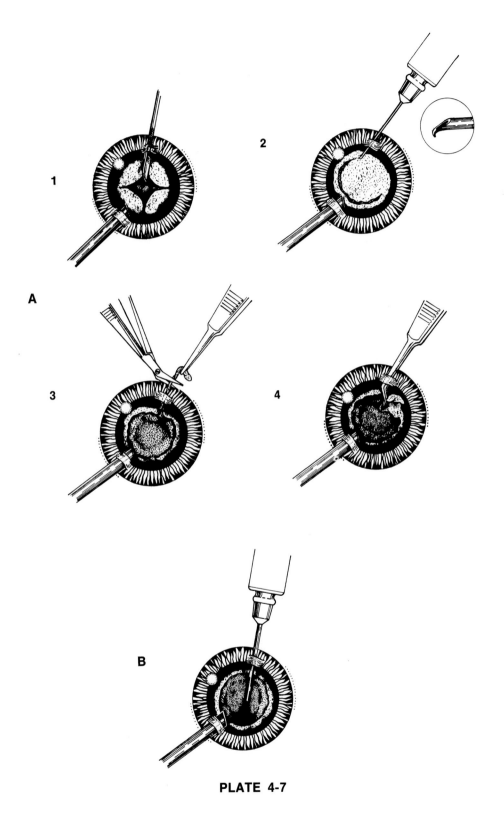

A

1

2

3

4

B

PLATE 4-7

PLATE 4-8

A Rarely, the lens material cannot be aspirated completely from the superior 12 o'clock position. The irrigating cannula then is removed from the 7 o'clock position and placed into the superior incision, the microscope is shifted laterally, and the aspirating needle is placed into the former irrigation incision at the 7 o'clock position. Aspiration of the remaining lens material is then carried out.

The posterior capsule then is examined carefully. At this time, a decision is made whether or not to fenestrate this capsule. In about 80% of cases, even when the posterior capsule remains clear at the end of the procedure, a secondary membrane that requires a second procedure will develop. Polishing the posterior capsule is not entirely effective in the long term because of the exuberant growth of anterior capsule cells from the periphery in many cases. The recent trend is to be more vigorous about fenestrating the posterior capsule even when it appears to be completely clear. An attempt is made to avoid the vitreous face. If vitreous is lost, an anterior vitrectomy is done with a suction cutting instrument.

B In cases in which an opacity of the posterior capsule remains after aspiration of the lens, this opacity must be removed in order for the procedure to be optically successful. This may be done with a needle knife or with a cystitome by carefully placing the tip of the instrument through the capsule and then tearing the capsule while avoiding the hyaloid face. This can be done if care is taken to avoid thrusting the instrument into the vitreous. Small tears may be enlarged by careful use of a cyclodialysis spatula.

C The posterior capsule may be chopped and aspirated with the Ocutome tip. In these cases the anterior hyaloid face invariably ruptures, and an anterior vitrectomy must be done.

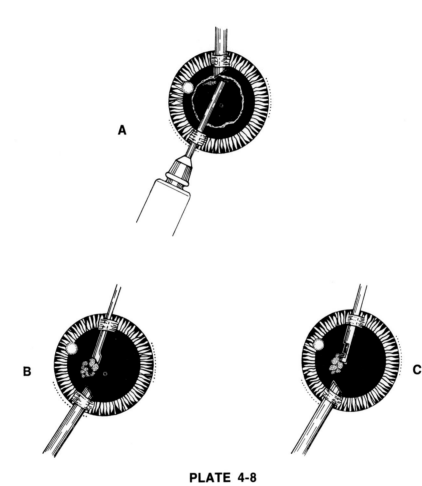

A

B

C

PLATE 4-8

PLATE 4-9

A Vitreous may enter the anterior chamber after the hyaloid face ruptures.

B In this event the Ocutome is used to do a shallow, anterior vitrectomy.

C Before use of the Ocutome, cellulose acetate sponges were used to bring the vitreous up to the wound, excise it, and vitreous was swept clear from the wound with a Barraquer cyclodialysis spatula.

D The vitreous, however, has a tendency to follow the spatula out of the eye and in spite of the surgeon's best efforts, one of the incisions is likely to have a vitreous adhesion. Anterior vitrectomy through the corneal incision reduces this likelihood.

E A moderate-size air bubble is then placed into the anterior chamber and the incisions are closed. Suture material is usually 8-0 collagen, but 9-0 or 10-0 Ethilon may be used. In about one third of cases, one or both corneal incisions are left unsutured.

F It is important that the air bubble in the anterior chamber not be too large. An excessively large air bubble may lead to the formation of peripheral anterior synechiae, because the bubble tends to assume a spherical shape, pressing central iris posteriorly and bringing peripheral iris forward. Iridectomies are not routinely done but should be done if inflammation is present or suspected. The pupil should be kept dilated for several weeks.

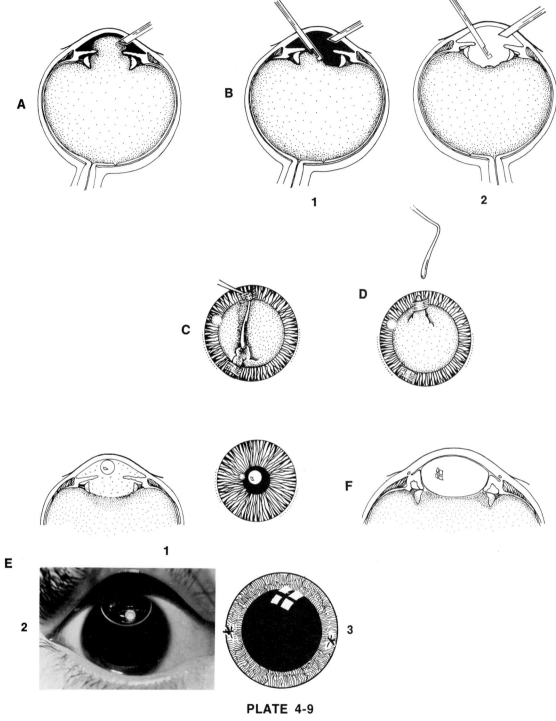

PLATE 4-9

Traumatic cataract with occlusiopupillae

When an ectopic pupil is present because of trauma or congenital causes, an iridectomy to allow a central visual access may be performed. In cases of rubella cataracts, a sector iridectomy and several sphincterotomies inferiorly are performed. Optical iridectomies in place of cataract surgery are seldom if ever indicated for children.

Postoperatively, patients are treated with atropine, 0.5% drops, twice a day and sodium sulfacetamide, 10% drops, twice a day for 5 days. After this, the atropine is continued for 8 weeks or longer, depending on the anterior chamber reaction. In cases of traumatic or otherwise complicated cataracts or cases in which inflammation is present, 2 mg of dexamethasone is injected subconjunctivally postoperatively. The eye is patched, and a shield may or may not be used. The patch is removed in 12 to 24 hours, and the patients are discharged the day following surgery. We require that patients be seen on a daily basis for the first 5 days postoperatively.

Removal of fibrous membranes

When a fibrous membrane is encountered, either after an uncomplicated cataract discission and aspiration or after injury, special techniques are required. These membranes are extremely tough and resistant to cutting because they "give" when a knife is drawn against them. Scissors are ideal for cutting these membranes, but scissors require a much larger incision to be effective and can be unwieldy under these circumstances. An alternative method of removing these dense membranes is the use of a mechanical device such as the Ocutome. The Ocutome works in a guillotinelike manner. Material is drawn into the opening port and then chopped by a reciprocating, pistonlike knife. Anterior chamber infusion is maintained through a separate port in a similar manner to the standard discission and aspiration technique.

PLATE 4-10

A Updrawn pupil with a dense membranous cataract and anterior synechiae.

B A sharp needle knife (McCaslin) is used to separate the anterior synechiae and then to fenestrate the membranous cataract.

C The Ocutome is placed in the anterior chamber with the tip through the hole in the cataractous membrane. The to-and-fro cutting piston nibbles away the cataract and enlarges the pupil. Gentle suction of 3 to 5 pounds per square inch is employed.

D The pupil may be enlarged with a very regular border using this technique.

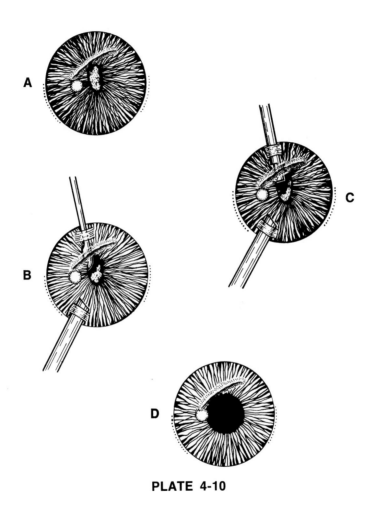

PLATE 4-10

Subluxated lenses

Subluxated lenses have been reported in Marfan syndrome, homocystinuria, syphilis after trauma, and with sulphite oxidase deficiency or hyperlysinemia. These lenses should be removed when they produce a significant visual impairment for the patient or when the persistence of such a lens poses a threat to the patient's eye as with anterior subluxation and pupillary block. Retention of a subluxated lens causes the patient to endure extreme myopia with astigmatism or aphakia. In general, if a subluxated lens is to be removed, it is better to do so while some zonular fibers remain intact and the lens is tethered within the pupillary zone.

The technique for discission and aspiration of a subluxated lens follows. The patient is prepared as for a discission and aspiration of an infantile cataract. The irrigating needle is placed through clear cornea at the point coincident with the direction and extent of the greatest lens subluxation. At a point 180° from this, the anterior chamber is entered with the discission knife and a 3-mm opening is made in the lens capsule, just anterior to the equater. A 22-gauge end aspirating Gass needle is then placed into the intracapsular substance of the lens, and the lens material is gently aspirated. Every attempt is made to remove as much of this material as possible with a single entry into the lens capsule. This may be accomplished by changing the barrel of the aspirating instrument or by having a separate exhaust port and a double-barreled needle.

When the lens material has been aspirated completely, a fine von Mondach forceps is used to grasp the lens capsule, and this is "teased" out of the incision, or the Ocutome is used to cut and remove the capsule and attached vitreous. Incisions are closed in a manner described for cataract. The patient is followed postoperatively in a similar manner to patients who undergo discission and aspiration.

PLATE 4-11

A After a chamber-forming needle has been placed, a 1.5-mm incision is made in clear cornea, a small (2.0- to 3.0-mm) incision is made in the lens capsule, and a 22-gauge Gass aspirating needle is placed into the lens cortex.

B Steady aspiration is carried out with an attempt to obtain all the intracapsular material without removing the needle.

C As aspiration continues, the capsule collapses.

D When the intracapsular contents are aspirated, the capsule is teased out with fine forceps.

E The Ocutome is used to remove any remaining lens material and to perform an anterior vitrectomy.

F The postoperative course usually includes more inflammatory response requiring pupillary dilatation for 10 weeks with 0.5% atropine and topical corticosteroid drops.

94

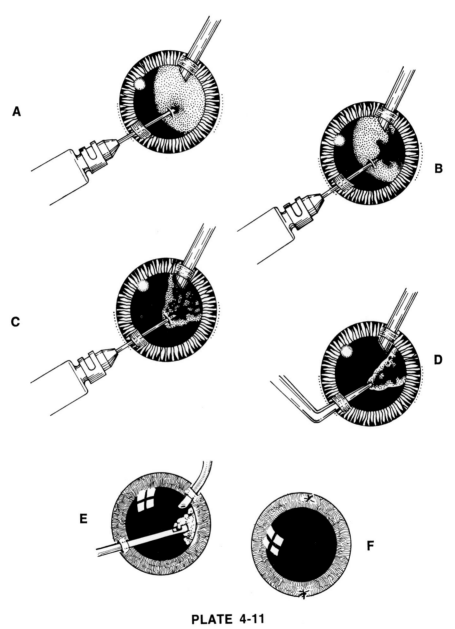

PLATE 4-11

95

OPTICAL CORRECTION OF THE APHAKIC INFANT

Contact lenses are fitted using the "too steep" technique. Contact lens fitting may be done preoperatively. To do this, when the patient is brought to the operating room, a trial contact lens is placed on the eye and fluorescein stain is placed in the cul-de-sac between the cornea and the posterior surface of the lens. A steep lens of approximately 7.0 mm central posterior curve or less is used initially. This lens ordinarily produces an air bubble. Lenses of decreasing steepness are then applied to the cornea until the bubble just disappears. If the ideal fit has been passed, a dark spot will appear centrally indicating that the lens is too flat and that no fluorescein is under the lens centrally. Going to a slightly flatter lens than the last one that produces a bubble or a slightly steeper lens than the last one that produces the dark central spot produces a satisfactory fit. We have found this to be more accurate and more practical than use of a keratometer in infants.

After the cataract is removed and the corneal sutures are out, an aphakic lens of the appropriate dimension is placed on the eye under topical anesthesia. It is possible to perform retinoscopy in the clinic or in a pediatric anesthesia clinic about 2 weeks postoperatively. Lenses of appropriate power are then prescribed. When contact lenses cannot be worn, spectacles are prescribed. We ordinarily prescribe approximately 2.5 to 3.0 D more plus corrections than indicated by the refraction. Hard contact lenses have been more satisfactory than soft lenses because they are more manageable for parents and are cheaper. The increased comfort of a soft lens has no real advantage for children, because it is the insertion and removal that causes parents difficulty, not the time of infant tolerance of the lens. Extended wear soft lenses, although not approved, are being attempted in experimental situations and may prove to be the most practical treatment.

PLATE 4-12

A A contact lens with a central posterior curve of 6.80 mm is too steep, as indicated by the bubble pattern in the fluorescein layer between the cornea and the posterior surface of the lens.

B A contact lens with a posterior central curve of 7.20 mm is too flat, as indicated by the lack of fluorescein between the cornea and the posterior curve of the lens.

C A contact lens with a posterior central curve of 7.05 mm is just right, as indicated by the even layer of fluorescein between the cornea and the posterior surface of the lens.

D A bilaterally aphakic 3-year-old boy wears single-vision aphakic spectacles.

E A 4-year-old boy with bilateral aphakia wears contact lenses.

Too steep

Too flat

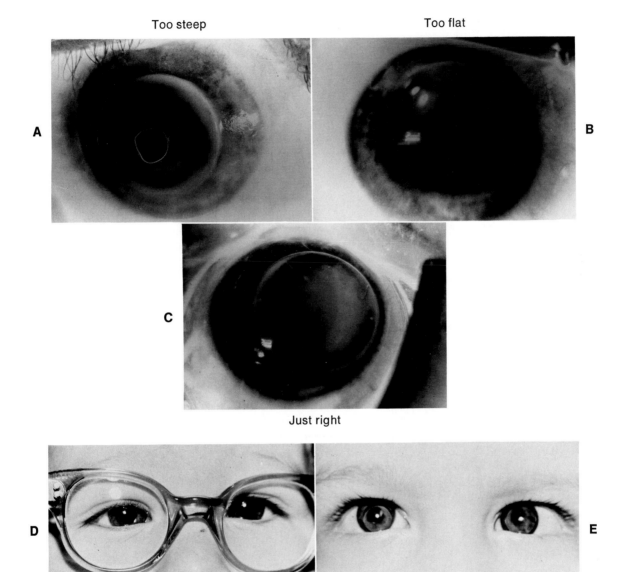

A

B

C

Just right

D

E

PLATE 4-12

One of the most discouraging and frustrating parts of the management of infantile cataracts is the use of a contact lens in a unilateral cataract, combined with patching of the good eye. In our experience, 20/80 vision has been the best obtained from an otherwise successful early operated unilateral cataract. Others have claimed better success, but even the successful cases are few and far between and stand out only as unusual examples rather than comprising a significant percentage of the infantile cataract surgeon's results.

Bilateral cataracts are treated satisfactorily with glasses and unless the parents wish otherwise, patients are given glasses until they are old enough to be responsible contact lens wearers.

Intraocular lenses have been placed in children's eyes by a few surgeons, but this practice has not gained general acceptance. Reported good results such as 20/40 vision in a unilateral congenital cataract operated on at age 5 are so contrary to all other published data that they stand out as unusual occurrences. That an infant's eye can withstand the implantation of a lens at least for a few years is undeniable, but the inaccuracy of this optical correction, pigment deposition on the lens, intraocular inflammation, uncertainties about the long-term tolerance of an intraocular foreign body, and lack of convincing evidence that visual results are improved over those obtained by the use of contact lenses and/or spectacles suggests that prudence be used in recommending intraocular lenses for children.

Complications encountered with congenital cataract surgery are extremely rare in spite of the fact that routine iridectomies are not done, and we have only rarely encountered postoperative glaucoma or flat chambers. We have seen no cases of endophthalmitis following cataract extraction and no uncomplicated infantile cataract patients have suffered retinal detachment. We have seen retinal detachment occur in a patient after cataract extraction for a subluxated lens and in one patient after discission and aspiration of a traumatic cataract.

Chapter 5

THE NASOLACRIMAL SYSTEM

Congenital obstruction of the nasolacrimal drainage system is a common condition that is symptomatic in approximately 2% of infants. This obstruction usually results from a membrane (valve of Hasner) at the distal portion of the nasolacrimal duct. This obstruction resolves spontaneously in the majority of cases. In other cases, massage and time, with or without antibiotics, seem to resolve the issue.

Occasionally, however, obstruction persists and intervention of a mechanical nature is required. While the usual obstruction is membranous, in more severe cases the entire bony canal may be underdeveloped or misdirected. Maldevelopment of the proximal portion of the system may occur but is less common. Some infants may be born with a distended nasolacrimal sac that results in a secondary closure of the valve of Rosenmuller, where the common canaliculi enter the nasolacrimal sac. The rather acute angle here is easily compromised further by swelling of the sac. Gentle massage may empty the sac through the puncta or though the nasolacrimal duct into the nose; when this can be accomplished it usually is curative. Often, however, the distended sac cannot be relieved by massage. In those cases, infection is the inevitable result if a successful probing is not carried out.

When the sac becomes infected (dacryocystitis), spontaneous drainage through the skin or spread of the infection to contiguous structures may occur. Systemic and topical antibiotics and surgical drainage of the abcess cavity are indicated in such instances. Surgical drainage may be accomplished by a stab wound incision through the skin over the abcess or by a keratome-type incision at the medial canthus on the conjunctival surface deep to the canaliculi and extending into the sac. This incision allows drainage into the palpebral fissure but does not leave a visible scar. Once the inflammatory process has subsided, the original obstruction site must be relieved either by probing or by probing supplemented by intubation of the system with silicone tubing.

Parents will bring their child to the ophthalmologist originally with the complaint that epiphora is occurring or that the eye "matters." This may not be obvious to the examiner on casual inspection if the infant is in an air-conditioned room and is not crying. However, in most cases the eye can be seen to be wet on close observation, and examination with a magnifier such as loupes will demonstrate an increased lacrimal lake. If any doubt about lacrimal obstruction remains, fluorescein should be instilled into both cul-de-sacs. It will disappear rapidly from the normal side but will persist on the obstructed side.

Frequently, the child will have had several courses of topical medication and massage supervised by his pediatrician, which is the appropriate initial treatment. If this has been the case, one may proceed with nasolacrimal duct probing. With a child less than 6 months of age, probing can be done in the office. The child is mummified, topical anesthesia is instilled in the cul-de-sac, the puncta are dilated, and a Bowman probe is passed through the system. The probe should be allowed to find its own course through the upper system, with no force being used except in the nasolacrimal duct. Only rarely are lacrimal obstructions encountered in the canaliculi in young patients.

Attempts to force the probe through such "obstructions" generally result in perforation of the canaliculi in small children. Bowman probe sizes 000 and 00 are most satisfactory. Too large a probe can rupture the canaliculus from the puncta or strip the epithelium from the canaliculus, resulting in a stricture that is more significant than the original distal obstruction.

TABLE 1. Treatment scheme for infantile nasolacrimal drainage system obstruction

Classification presentation	Treatment
1. Epiphora, no infection	Massage and time
2. Epiphora, with infection	Massage, 10% sodium sulfacetamide gtts topically. Culture when necessary
3. Epiphora, with or without infection persisting after two treatment courses as noted in 1 or 2 above	Probe system with 000 or 00 Bowman probe; patient awake, if less than 6 mos; with anesthesia if older than 6 mos
4. Epiphora, with or without infection persisting after two or more probings of the nasolacrimal system	Intubation of system with silicone tubing; leave in place for 4 weeks to 4 months; rule out abnormal nasal anatomy; fracture turbinate if necessary
5. Persistent lacrimal duct obstruction	Repeat step 4 or proceed with dacryocystorhinostomy (generally not done in patients younger than 5 or 6 years if it can be avoided)
6. Persistent common canalicular obstruction	Conjunctival dacryocysto-rhinostomy
7. Acute dacryocystitis or amniotocele	Massage; topical and systemic antibiotics
8. Persistent dacryocystitis or amniotocele	Stab incision; topical and systemic antibiotics

PLATE 5-1

A The components of the nasolacrimal drainage system.
B Important dimensions of the nasolacrimal drainage system.

A single probing is curative in the majority of cases of nasolacrimal obstruction. In those cases in which an initial probing is not curative, the surgeon often can anticipate failure at the initial effort because of peculiarities in the anatomy. In these instances, repeat efforts at probing can be avoided, proceeding to early intubation of the system. In all instances, the presence of the probe in the nose should be verified by direct vision or by feeling the probe in the proper position with a second probe or instrument placed in the nose. Although one cannot be certain that the probe has emerged in the nose through the valve of Hasner without direct visualization, it is often not possible or practical to attempt direct visualization, particularly in an office setting.

Topical sodium sulfacetamide, 10% is given for a few days after probing. If the probing is curative, no further treatment is indicated. If not, repeat probing or intubation is indicated. If the child is over 6 months of age, we prefer to do the probing with the patient under general anesthesia. If endotracheal anesthesia is established for this procedure, irrigation may be done, but no irrigation is done if only a mask is used for anesthesia because of the risks of aspiration pneumonia.

Anomalies of the system may include absent puncta. Occasionally the puncta can be seen beneath the epithelium with a microscope. Punctal surgery with a stint such as a Veirs rod or a silicone tubing may be curative in such cases. In rare cases, a dacryocystostomy incision may permit retrograde probing for catheterization of the canaliculi. This should not be undertaken unless one is prepared to proceed with conjunctival dacryocystorhinostomy in case the retrograde efforts are unsuccessful.

ANATOMY OF THE NASOLACRIMAL SYSTEM

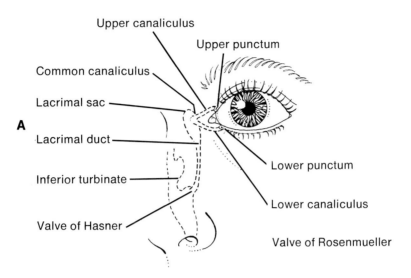

Upper canaliculus

Upper punctum

Common canaliculus

Lacrimal sac

A

Lacrimal duct

Inferior turbinate

Valve of Hasner

Lower punctum

Lower canaliculus

Valve of Rosenmueller

DIMENSIONS OF THE NASOLACRIMAL SYSTEM

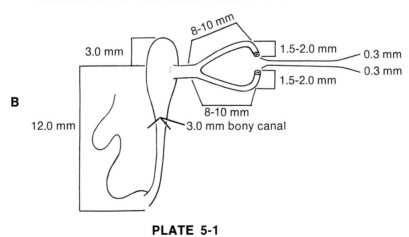

8-10 mm

3.0 mm

1.5-2.0 mm

0.3 mm

0.3 mm

1.5-2.0 mm

B

8-10 mm

12.0 mm

3.0 mm bony canal

PLATE 5-1

103

TECHNIQUE FOR PROBING THE NASOLACRIMAL SYSTEM

PLATE 5-2

A After the infant or child has been adequately mummified, sedated, or anesthetized, the puncta inferior and superior are dilated with a sterile, large, blunted safety pin. It should be remembered that the vertical portion of the canaliculus is only 1.5 to 2.0 mm. If the pin is pushed in farther it should be directed in a medial direction.

B A Bowman probe 000 or 00 is then inserted vertically into the dilated punctum.

C After passing 1.5 to 2.0 mm vertically, the probe is directed in a medial direction gently until a distinct bony feeling is encountered. The probe will travel approximately 12 to 14 mm before hitting this bony surface, which is the medial wall of the lacrimal sac adjacent to the wall of the lacrimal fossa.

D The Bowman probe is then raised vertically while the tip remains in contact with the medial wall of the sac.

E When the entrance to the lacrimal duct is encountered, the probe is directed straight downward to 15° posteriorly for 12 to 15 mm. At this point, some obstruction may be encountered. The probe should stop when it encounters the floor of the nasal cavity.

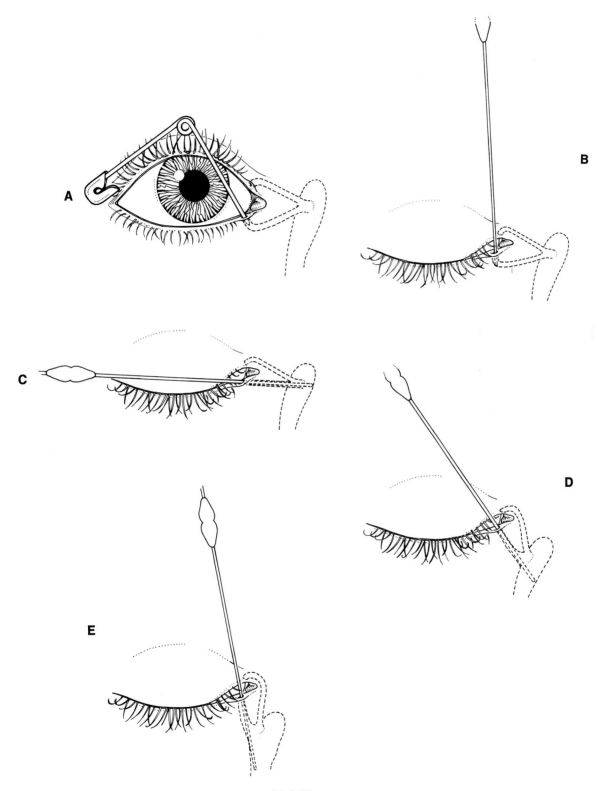

PLATE 5-2

PLATE 5-3

When the probe enters the nose or is thought to have entered the nose, its presence can be confirmed in two ways. It can be observed by using a speculum and head light, or it can be felt by touching it with a second probe placed in the nose. Our preference is to place a large probe in the nose and actually palpate and move the probe that has been passed through the system. This proves that this probe is in the nose, although without direct observation one cannot be sure that the probe has emerged through the proper orifice.

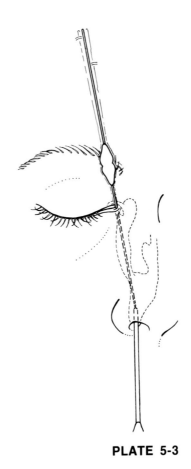

PLATE 5-3

Silicone tubing

In cases of chronic nasolacrimal system obstruction where a patent system has been demonstrated, silicone (Quickert-Dryden) tubes may be placed in the system and left in place from weeks to months. The average length of time that silicone tubes have been left in place by us is 3 months. We saw one case where tubes were in place for 18 months. The patients are universally comfortable with the tubes, but epiphora will be present to some degree. Silicone tubes are successful in approximately 70% of cases. When epiphora persists or recurs after the tubes are removed, they may be replaced. However, when the initial course of tube placement has been unsuccessful, secondary tube placement is less likely to relieve the epiphora. These patients may have a deficiency in the lacrimal pump mechanism (rare in children), or the nasolacrimal anatomy precludes the establishment of an effective drainage system. Since a failed silicone tube is followed by a dacryocystorhinostomy, every effort within reason is taken to secure success with probing or with intubation if this treatment is required.

Placement of silicone tube

PLATE 5-4

A A silicone tube of the smallest diameter possible is fitted over the end of a small-diameter wire Quickert tube. If the silicone is heated in a pan of warm water, it slips over the probe more readily. After the silicone tube has been fitted over approximately 20 mm of the probe, it is glued on with cyanoacrylate glue.

B After the nasolacrimal system has been probed with confirmation of the probe tip *in the nose,* the Quickert probe with silicone tube is placed in the system using the upper canaliculus. A right angle hook is used to direct the probe tip anteriorly toward the external nose. This usually puts a bend in the tube, which precludes withdrawal of the probe through the canaliculi.

C The anteriorly directed bent tip of the probe is grasped with a fine-tipped alligator forceps and is pulled out the nose.

D The probe is completely withdrawn from the nose with the silicone tube following. A slow, steady pull is employed to reduce the chance of the silicone tube slipping off the probe. When this happens, as it frequently does when the system is tight, the process must be repeated. A drop of mineral oil at the punctum may help lubricate passage of the silicone tube.

E The lower canaliculus is intubated in the same way.

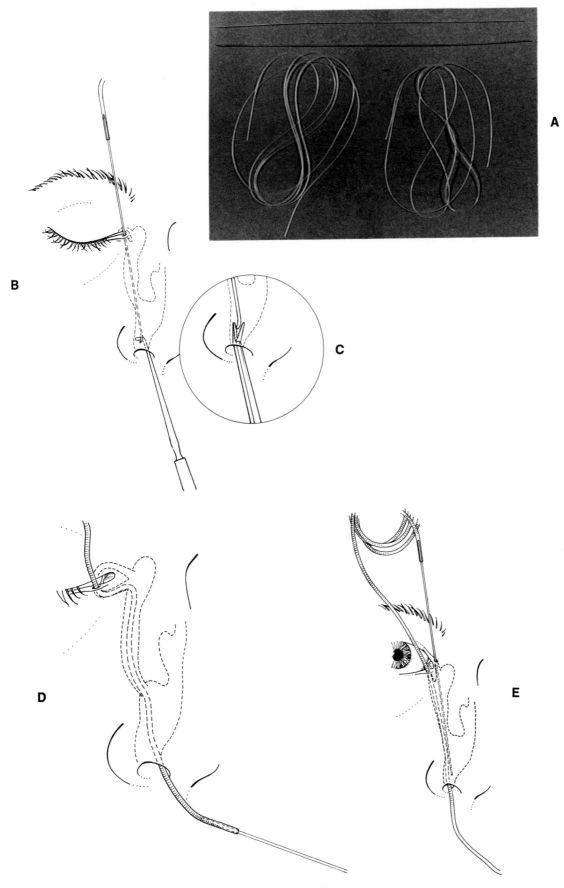

PLATE 5-4

PLATE 5-5

A When both silicone tubes have been withdrawn from the nose, from 10 to 12 overhand knots are placed to secure the ends.

B The mass of knots are placed posteriorly in the nasopharynx.

With the tubes in place, a sneeze may cause the knots in the silicone to become visible at the nostril. A simple "sniff" may get the tubes back in place or they may be replaced with a cotton-tipped applicator. The tubes are easily removed in the office in a cooperative patient. Younger children require a simple anesthetic such as might be administered for a probe. The technique for tube removal is to reach in the nose with a bayonet forceps to grasp the silicone tube, snip the silicone tube *between* the puncta, and then pull the tube completely out of the nose.

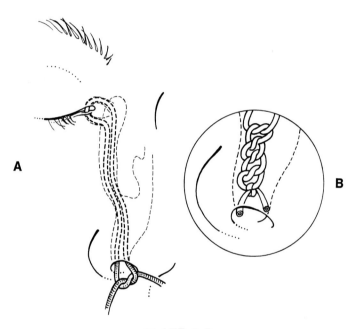

PLATE 5-5

Setup for probing nasolacrimal duct

PLATE 5-6

The setup for probing of the nasolacrimal duct includes these instruments:
Disposable 2 cc syringe filled with fluorescein-dyed saline solution
Nasolacrimal duct cannula, 23 and 25 gauge
Safety pin punctum dilator
Cotton-tipped applicator
Assorted Bowman probes, No. 000 to 2
Stapes hook
Nasal speculum
Gauge, 4 × 4

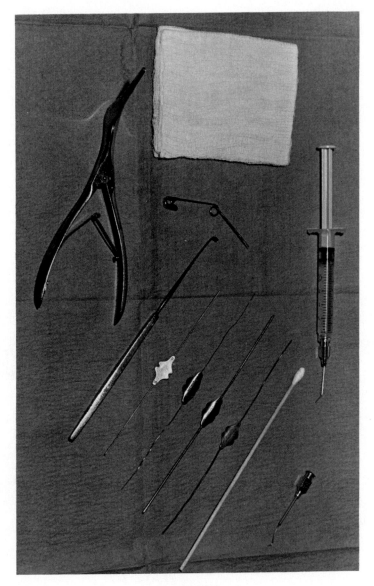

PLATE 5-6

Setup for placement of silicone tube

PLATE 5-7

The setup for placement of the silicone tube includes these instruments:
Atomizer
Neo-Synephrine, 0.25% solution
Suction probe
Glue
Alligator forceps
No. 15 Bard-Parker blade
Safety pin punctum dilator
Bowman probe
Quickert probes, assorted sizes
Assorted small diameter silicone tubes
Cotton-tip applicators
Nasal speculum
Stapes hook
Hemostat
Sharp-pointed scissors

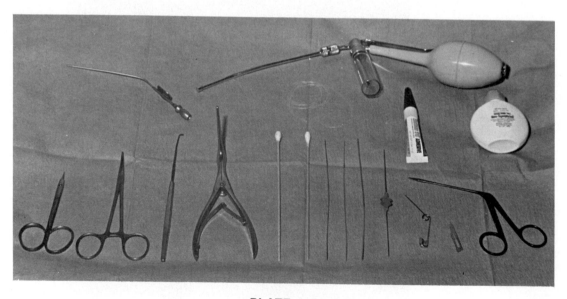

PLATE 5-7

114

DACRYOCYSTORHINOSTOMY

Dacryocystorhinostomy (DCR) is effective in children with patent canaliculi but should be reserved, if possible, for children over 5 or 6 years of age in whom more conservative measures have failed. If the canaliculi are *not* functioning, a conjunctival DCR is the only alternative to constant epiphora. The care that these tubes require dictates that each case must be selected on the basis of the surgeon's assessment of the particular patient's suitability, not only for the procedure but for follow-up care as well.

Dacryocystorhinostomy is performed with the usual techniques. An attempt is made to avoid the angular vessels either by bringing the incision medial or lateral to these vessels, which are found 4 to 6 mm medial to the medial canthus. The incision is carried down to the periosteum, which is then incised with a scalpel. Periosteum is reflected temporally with a Freer elevator. When the lacrimal fossa has been exposed and the periosteum and sac are reflected temporally, an opening into the nose is made that straddles the anterior lacrimal crest. This incision may be made with a Stryker saw or a chisel and mallet, but it is usually enlarged with a Kerasen punch. The bony opening should be at least 20 mm long and 15 mm wide. A probe is placed in the upper or lower canaliculus and directed medially until its tip is visible indenting the nasal wall of the lacrimal sac. At this point, the wall of the lacrimal sac is incised in an H shape forming an anterior and posterior flap. A similar incision is made in the mucous membrane of the nose. The sac and mucosal posterior flaps are secured to one another with absorbable suture. A No. 14 French catheter is directed into the nose, through the bony ostium, and into the fundus of the sac, where it is sutured in place with a 4-0 catgut suture. The anterior flaps are then secured with absorbable suture. The catheter is sutured to the external nose with a 5-0 black silk suture tied over a small rubber peg. After 10 days the silk suture is removed and the catheter pulled free. This is followed by irrigation if the child is cooperative.

A silicone tube through the canaliculi may be used at the same time as the DCR, with the tube threaded through the catheter. When the catheter is pulled, it is slipped over the silicone tubes, which are then left in place for several weeks or months. In this instance the tubes are emerging in the nose through the DCR opening, not through the nasolcarimal duct.

Ectopic puncta may be associated with obstruction of the nasolacrimal system. In this instance the ectopic puncta should be excised, preferably down to their exit from the normal part of the system, and the entirety of the redundant system should be excised. Fulgurating the ectopic punctum will not be effective.

PLATE 5-8

A The incision for dacryocystorhinostomy is carried down to the periosteum, which is then incised with a scalpel.

B The Freer elevator is used to reflect periosteum temporally so that an opening into the nose can be made.

C After the bony opening is made, the probe is placed in the canaliculus and directed medially until the tip is visible, indenting the nasal wall of the lacrimal sac.

D Anterior and posterior flaps are formed by incising the walls of the lacrimal sac and mucous membrane of the nose in an H shape. An absorbable suture secures the sac and mucosal posterior flaps to one another.

E A No. 14 French catheter is sutured to the fundus of the sac with a 4-0 catgut suture, and the anterior flaps are secured with absorbable suture.

F The catheter has been secured to the external nose with a 5-0 silk suture tied over a small rubber peg.

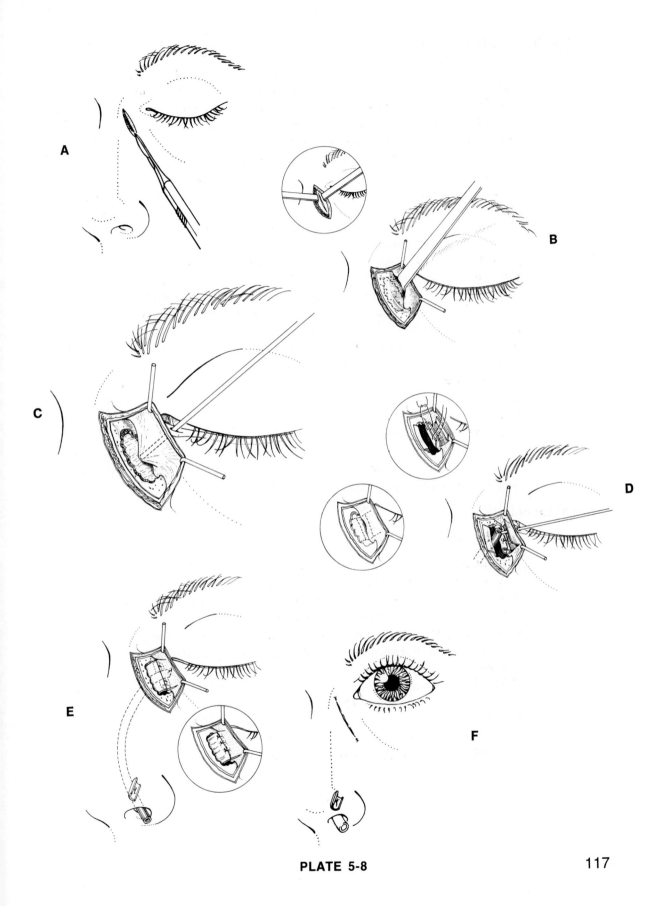

PLATE 5-8

117

CONJUNCTIVORHINOSTOMY

In cases in which epiphora results from obstruction of the upper or proximal nasolacrimal drainage system, conjunctivorhinostomy is employed. This procedure joins the lacrimal lake to the inside of the nose with the help of a silicone or Pyrex tube. Conjunctivorhinostomy is the least physiologic of the procedures to relieve epiphora and is the most difficult to maintain, although it should succeed in virtually all cases if enough effort is expended by the physician and the patient.

The procedure employs a 15-to 20-mm window in bone straddling the lacrimal crest identical to that employed with the dacryocystorhinostomy. A stab incision is then made beginning just temporal to the caruncle, passing through the conjunctiva and deeper tissues and through the bony window. A polyethylene tube that has had a Reinecke tube placed over it is placed through the stab incision and is brought out through the nose. The polyethylene tube is pulled through until the Reinecke tube is seated, and then the polyethylene tube is removed. The deep tissues and skin incision are closed, and a nonabsorbable suture is used to anchor the flange of the Reinecke tube deep in the lacrimal lake. Instead of a Reinecke tube, a Jones tube may be used. If a Reinecke tube is used initially, it may be replaced with a Jones Pyrex tube later. In a few cases, after several years of use, the tube may be removed with continued patency and function of the tract. Toilet of the tube can be accomplished by the patient employing the Valsalva maneuver. The principal complication of the conjunctivorhinostomy tube is the formation of granulation tissue around the tube opening. This requires careful excision of tissue and sometimes repositioning of the tube. Silicone tubes appear to be more prone to produce granulation tissue than the Pyrex tube.

Surgical technique

PLATE 5-9

A An incision is made in a manner similar to that for a DCR, and a bony window is made at the anterior lacrimal crest.

B Sharp-pointed scissors are thrust through at the caruncle and lacrimal sac until the tips are exposed in the wound.

C A polyethylene tube is passed up the nose, through the bony window, and is engaged with a hemostat that has been placed in the path made by the scissors in step B.

D The polyethylene tube is pulled out through the conjunctival incision, and the Reinecke tube is threaded.

E The polyethylene tube is pulled out the nose, seating the Reinecke tube, which is sutured in the lacrimal lake area with 5.0 merseline.

F The Reinecke tube may be replaced with a Pyrex Jones tube later.

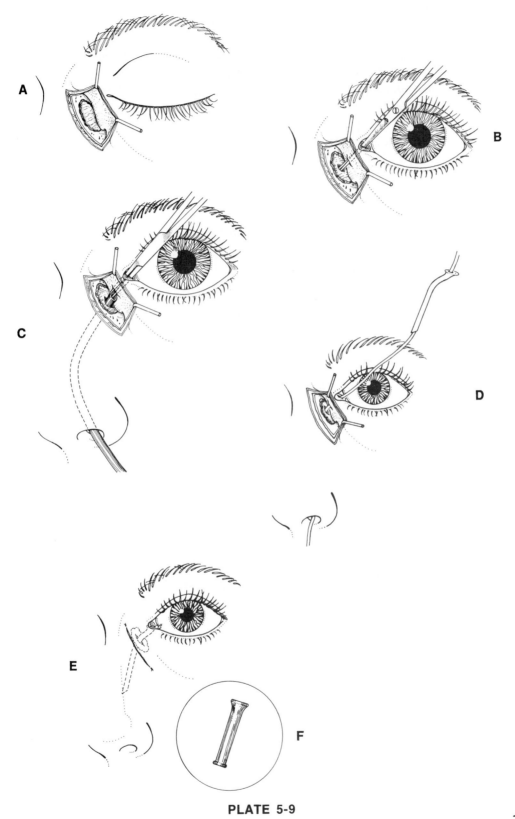

PLATE 5-9

119

CASE HISTORIES

PLATE 5-10

A This infant demonstrates severe dacryocystitis. Pressure over the distended sac produced a moderate amount of purulent material.

B Since the sac remained distended after palpation, the abcess was drained by means of an incision through skin over the sac. This incision heals rapidly and without a significant scar. Both systemic and topical antibiotics should be used in cases with acute dacryocystitis whether drainage is employed or not.

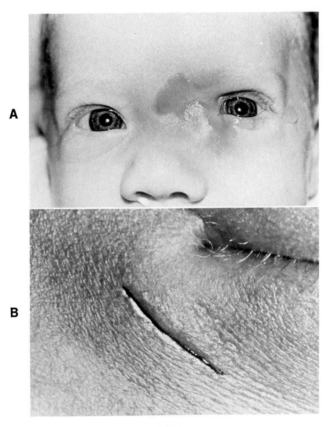

PLATE 5-10

PLATE 5-11

A Typical "wet eye" appearance of lacrimal obstruction in an infant. No infection is present. Often, mothers clean such an eye before bringing their child in for examination, making diagnosis more difficult.

B A tell-tale sign of chronic lacrimal obstruction is the matted appearance of the lashes in the eye with the obstruction. The right eye is affected.

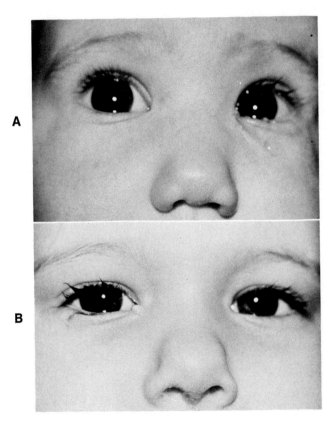

A

B

PLATE 5-11

123

PLATE 5-12

A Bilateral chronic lacrimal obstruction in a 3-year-old girl. Bilateral conjunctivitis is present.

B Severe dacryocystitis in a 6-year-old girl. The infection has spread to the preseptal area.

C Acute dacryocystitis after spontaneous rupture of the abscess.

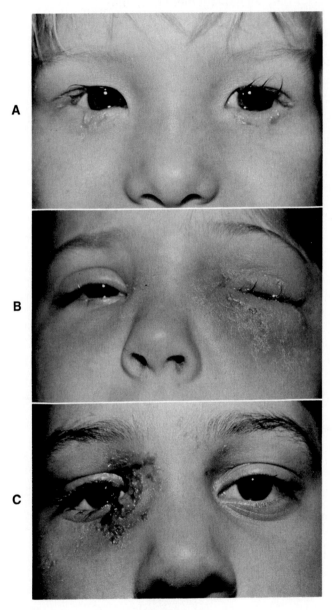

PLATE 5-12

PLATE 5-13

A A severed lower canaliculus has been reapproximated over a stint that has been placed through both upper and lower system.

B An 11-year-old boy has a Reinecke tube in place. Granuloma formation of the conjunctiva over the tube opening in the lacrimal lake presents a significant management problem.

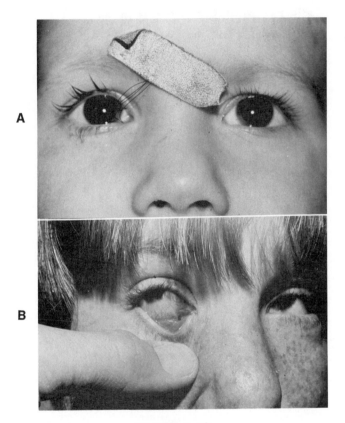

PLATE 5-13

Chapter 6

GLAUCOMA

Glaucoma is a rare congenital anomaly and relatively uncommon as an acquired childhood disease. Glaucoma occurring in children differs greatly from glaucoma in adults from the standpoints of incidence, diagnosis, medical and surgical treatment, and prognosis.

GENERAL CONSIDERATIONS
Incidence

Congenital (infantile) glaucoma occurs in approximately 1 in 25,000 births, being slightly less common than sporadic retinoblastoma. Other types of glaucoma occurring secondarily as a part of congenital ocular abnormalities, such as Sturge-Weber syndrome, aniridia, and mesodermal dysgenesis, are also uncommon. Acquired childhood glaucoma can result from a variety of precursors, including trauma, inflammation, tumors, postsurgical insult, and unknown, idiopathic causes. Although this type of glaucoma is also relatively uncommon, acquired glaucoma is seen more often than the congenital variety.

Diagnosis

Congenital (infantile) glaucoma is characterized by epiphora, photophobia, and blepharospasm in an infant with large, usually hazy corneas present at birth or developing during the first year of life. The diagnosis must be confirmed at an examination with the patient anesthetized, which includes determination of intraocular pressure, measurement of corneal diameter, gonioscopic evaluation of the anterior chamber angle, and careful study of the optic nerve head of each eye. Other acquired childhood glaucoma is diagnosed by measurement of the intraocular pressure during an examination with the patient anesthetized or, when possible, while the child is awake. Some acquired glaucomas are suspected on the basis of a coexisting ocular abnormality that has a known predilection to cause glaucoma. Childhood glaucoma follow-up includes intraocular pressure checks and observation of the optic nerve head. Visual field examinations are usually not done accurately and, therefore, are not useful in children under 5 or 6 years of age.

Treatment

Congenital glaucoma is treated surgically with goniotomy (one to three in each eye) or, if that fails, with a filtering procedure. Medical therapy in the form of topical agents that decrease aqueous production or increase its outflow are useful but not as effective as they usually are in adults. Systemically administered carbonic anhydrase inhibitors lower intraocular pressure effectively in children and are relatively free from side effects in appropriate doses. Acquired glaucoma is treated medically or surgically according to the pathologic condition present and the special needs of each patient.

Prognosis

The overall prognosis for congenital (infantile) glaucoma is relatively good if the condition is diagnosed early and if goniotomy is done and repeated if necessary until intraocular pressure is reduced to normal. In unilateral cases, careful refraction must be done, optical correction should be provided, and possibly patching should be done so that anisometropic amblyopia will not ensue. However, any type of childhood glaucoma has a guarded prognosis, because the long duration of the disease with the potential for a change in aqueous dynamics keeps optic nerve function in jeopardy. As with the adult disease, glaucoma in childhood, whether congenital or acquired, requires lifelong, diligent follow-up with timely, appropriate treatment.

PLATE 6-1

A The Shiøtz instrument is a valuable tool for the diagnosis of glaucoma in infants. It is usually used for intraocular pressure determination at an examination with the child anesthetized. The main advantages of the Shiøtz instrument are low cost, portability, and availability. With the Shiøtz instrument, lower intraocular pressure may be recorded in cases of decreased ocular rigidity.

B The portable applanation tonometer of Draeger or Perkins is a useful, accurate instrument for determining intraocular pressure in children. It may be used with the patient sitting up or supine. The problems associated with ocular rigidity are essentially eliminated with the applanation technique. The instrument is relatively expensive but portable. (The Draeger type is shown.)

C The standard clinical instrument for determining intraocular pressure is the Goldmann applanation tonometer. This provides an extremely accurate determination of intraocular pressure, obviating inaccuracies produced by altered ocular rigidity. However, it is difficult to obtain cooperation for this test in a child under 8 to 10 years of age.

D The Mackey-Marg instrument for determination of intraocular pressure is useful in cases of corneal irregularity or edema. The instrument produces a single tracing, which provides the instantaneous intraocular pressure reading.

E Another useful instrument for determining intraocular pressure in childhood glaucoma, in our experience, is the pneumatomograph. This instrument may be used with the patient sitting upright or supine. When the foot pedal is depressed, Freon inflates a thin-walled balloon at the tip of the testing probe. When the probe is placed against the eye, a sound is emitted, indicating that proper application of the instrument to the cornea has been obtained. A constant readout is recorded on heat-sensitive calibrated paper. Changes in the intraocular pressure associated with the pulse are readily detected and ensure that an accurate application is being maintained. We have found that the pneumatomograph provides pressure readings similar to or slightly higher than the Goldmann tonometer.

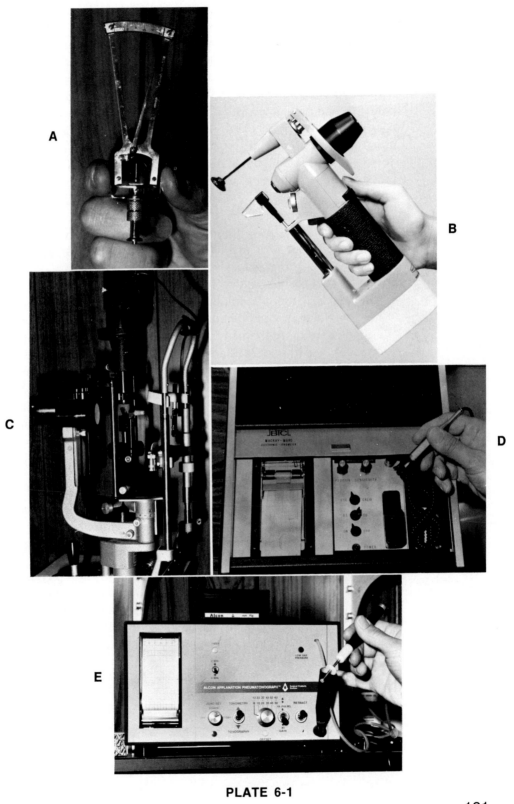

PLATE 6-1

Diagnostic techniques

Determining the intraocular pressure and evaluation of the optic nerve head are the most important tests in the diagnosis and follow-up of congenital or acquired childhood glaucoma. Normal intraocular pressure in infancy and childhood is between 10 and 20 mm Hg. However, children's eyes often can withstand intraocular pressure elevation to 30 mm Hg for considerable periods without significant insult to the optic nerve or visual function. It is our general policy to maintain intraocular pressures below 20 mm Hg in children when possible. However, in children with congenital glaucoma, we often follow pressures in the mid 20s without repeat of goniotomy provided the optic nerve appearance remains stable. The exact point where elevated intraocular pressure causes the need for glaucoma surgery cannot be dogmatically stated.

PLATE 6-2

A The typical patient with congenital (infantile) glaucoma has enlargement of one or both corneas. The cornea may be slightly hazy, epiphora is present, and photophobia is apparent.

B The normal corneal diameter in an infant is approximately 10.5 mm. At 1 year it is 11.5 mm, and in adulthood it is 12 mm or slightly more. The corneal diameters should be equal within 0.5 mm or less. A corneal diameter enlargement more than 1 mm over the exptected size should be cause for concern. The horizontal diameter is the one chosen for measurement.

C The increased intraocular pressure in congenital glaucoma causes corneal enlargement because the globe in the child under 6 months or 1 year of age is distensible. In the infant eye, the anterior portion of the globe stretches rather than the posterior. While the cornea is enlarging because of increased intraocular pressure, cracks or striae develop in Descemet's membrane. These are called Haab's striae and are usually horizontal or concentric and are 0.1 to 0.3 mm wide.

D The normal appearance of the infantile optic nerve head.

E A normal infantile optic nerve head demonstrating physiologic cupping.

F A moderate-size pathologic cup in a patient with congenital glaucoma.

G A severely cupped optic nerve resulting from congenital glaucoma.

Asymmetry of the cups in children occurs rarely as a physiologic phenomenon. When asymmetry exists, careful determination of the intraocular pressure should be carried out. In cases of adequately treated congenital glaucoma, Shaffer[42] has reported and we have observed a "filling in" of a cup several months after pressure was normalized.

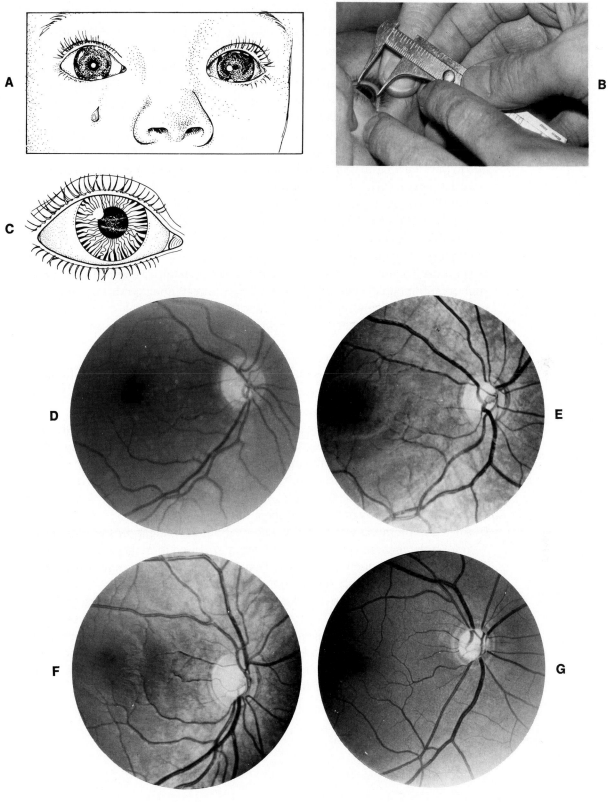

PLATE 6-2

Gonioscopy

Gonioscopy is an examination technique that allows direct observation of the anterior chamber angle. A Koeppe lens is used for examining the anterior chamber angle in a supine infant. Illumination and magnification can be obtained from a Barkan illuminator or by a fiberoptic head-mounted light source and magnifying loupes worn by the examiner. With the Koeppe lens, approximately 1/6 of a chamber angle can be viewed at a time. Because the lens is round, it is relatively easy to move around the patient and obtain a view of the entire angle in a relatively short time. A Koeppe lens may be placed on each eye to provide a rapid comparison of the chamber angles. Older, more cooperative patients may have gonioscopy performed while sitting at the biomicroscope. When this gonioscopy is done, a Goldmann three-mirror lens is used.

Study of the chamber angle is essential in childhood glaucomas. Readily observable chamber angle anomalies are frequently present, and in the case of infantile glaucoma, the prime treatment is a direct, surgical modification of the anterior chamber angle. Abnormalities of the chamber angle also occur in such infantile and childhood glaucomas as Sturge-Weber syndrome, aniridia, neurofibromatosis, mesodermal dysgenesis, and glaucomas resulting from trauma, intraocular surgery, or inflammatory conditions.

PLATE 6-3

A The three-mirror Goldmann lens provides an indirect view of the chamber angle. The test is performed usually with the patient sitting at the biomicroscope. A viscous gel is used between the lens and cornea.

B The Koeppe lens provides a direct view of the anterior chamber angle. Saline solution is used between the lens and cornea. This examination usually is done with the patient supine.

C The typical congenital glaucoma angle has a high inserting flat iris with an absent angle recess. Pectinate ligaments may be seen, as well as increased vascularity of the iris at the angle.

D After goniotomy, a white cleft is seen forming an angle recess. Scattered anterior synechiae with pigment clusters are seen in most postgoniotomy angles. These synechiae are usually sparse, and aqueous humor can ordinarily flow behind with access to the angle.

E Angle recession may be noted after severe contusion injury to the globe. A relatively deep white cleft is noted where the ciliary body has been separated from the scleral spur. The glaucoma that occurs after angle recession may occur months to years after the original injury. Yanoff* has suggested that the glaucoma results from the spread of a sheet of endothelial cells over the angle and onto the iris, shutting off the filtration process.

---

*Personal communication, December 1978.

F The anterior segment cleavage abnormality or mesodermal dysgenesis presents an extremely abnormal gonioscopic view. Multiple anterior synechiae and general lack of normal architecture are noted.

G Aniridia demonstrates a chamber angle with either no iris or a small remnant of iris. Sometimes this remnant can be anteriorly adherent, causing obstruction to the outflow channel. The equator of the lens and the zonular fibers are readily seen. Grant and Walton[14] have suggested prophylactic goniotomy in aniridia, but long-term results of this type of procedure are not known.

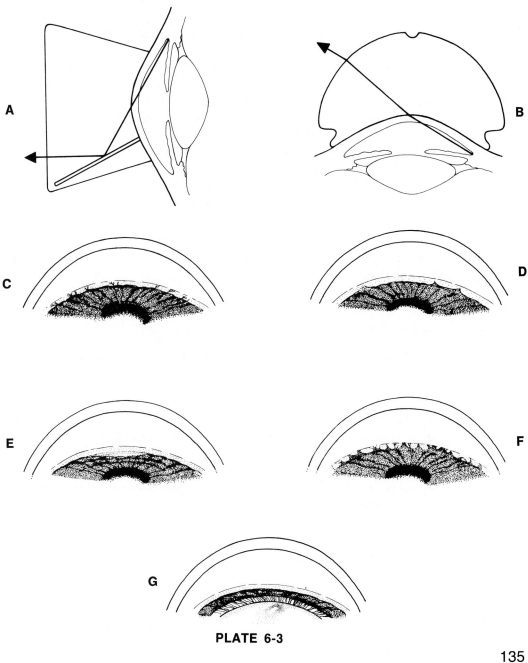

PLATE 6-3

TREATMENT
Infantile glaucoma (primary congenital glaucoma)

Infantile glaucoma becomes evident usually within the first few days, weeks, or months of life, occurring sporadically or as an autosomal recessive trait. It is characterized by corneal changes (either bilateral or unilateral), including enlargement, haziness, and horizontal striae (Haab's). The infant affected with glaucoma is photophobic and may have excess lacrimation. A differential diagnosis of striae includes birth trauma, congenital syphilis, and high myopia, all of which have normal intraocular pressure and normal-sized corneas. Excess lacrimation may be caused by inflammation, an obstructed lacrimal drainage system, or photophobia due to other causes such as albinism. Megalocornea may occur. This is often an inherited condition. The corneas are usually clear and appear to protrude with more curvature than do the enlarged corneas of congenital glaucoma. If a suspicion of congenital glaucoma exists, the child should be scheduled for examination under anesthesia. This includes evaluation of the following: corneal diameter, corneal integrity (edema, striae), the anterior chamber angle, and optic nerve head. The examination should take place in the operating room with the understanding that if glaucoma is diagnosed, a goniotomy will be performed. Goniotomy is not a difficult operation, but it does require extreme care. The lens must be avoided, and the goniotomy knife must be placed in the precise area superficial to the filtration meshwork, allowing the base of the iris to drop posteriorly as a result of the cutting of Barkan's membrane or the trabecular end of an abnormally placed meridional ciliary muscle (Maumenee). It is not a good idea to undertake this procedure without experience or careful preparation. Shaffer[42] has suggested that experience in goniotomy may be obtained by practicing on an anesthetized cat.

Goniotomy technique

PLATE 6-4

A Typical appearance of an infant with bilateral congenital glaucoma.

If a goniotomy is to be done, care should be taken to ensure the best possible view of the chamber angle. If the cornea is edematous and hazy, the epithelium should be removed with a No. 64 Beaver blade. The procedure can be done relatively easily, and the reepithelialization takes place rapidly in the infant.

Two basic techniques for performing a goniotomy are the Worst lens technique and the Barkan technique. Each of these techniques has the same goal, that is, reduction of intraocular pressure by increasing access of aqueous to the filtration network. Before goniotomy the pupil should be constricted with pilocarpine to provide protection for the lens.

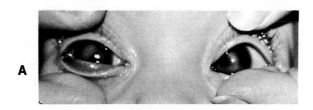

A

PLATE 6-4

PLATE 6-4—cont'd

B **(1)** The Worst technique employs a flanged goniotomy lens with an operating port, an infusion port, and four holes for securing the flange to the episclera. The lens may also have a fiberoptic light source (shown). Before goniotomy, the lens is sewn to conjunctiva with 4-0 or 5-0 silk sutures, and an 8-0 Vicryl suture is placed in a bridle manner to coincide with the operating port. This latter suture is used for countertraction when the goniotomy knife is thrust through the cornea to enter the anterior chamber. The traction suture must be removed and a separate suture used to close the operative site. Saline from a source a meter or so above the eye provides fluid between the lens and the cornea.

(2) The microscope is used for magnification and, if needed, illumination with the Worst technique. The Worst knife is a cannulated goniotomy knife that is attached to a saline-filled 20-cc syringe. This may be held above the patient to cause constant infusion for maintenance of the anterior chamber, or gentle pressure may be applied to the plunger by an assistant. Care should be taken not to apply too much pressure, because this will cause the cornea to become cloudy instantly.

(3) Initial goniotomy is carried out from a temporal corneal incision with goniotomy done in the nasal chamber angle. A No. 75 Beaver blade is used to cut down through cornea to Descemet's membrane. The cannulated Worst knife is then thrust into the anterior chamber, directed carefully across the anterior chamber just above the plane of the iris until the fibers of Barkan's membrane or whatever abnormality exists in front of the angle is encountered. The lens is stabilized by the operator.

(4) With the Barkan technique, a simple, dome-topped lens with one flattened side is used. This is placed on the cornea, and saline is placed between the cornea and lens. An assistant steadies the eye at the 6 and 12 o'clock positions usually by grasping the insertions of the superior and inferior rectus muscles with stout, locking forceps.

(5) The surgeon may use a fiberoptic head light for illumination and loupes for magnification or, preferably, the microscope may be used for illumination and magnification. The anterior chamber is entered with a tapered shaft Swann modification of the Barkan goniotomy knife. A No. 75 Beaver blade may be used to cut initially down to Descemet's membrane, or the entire incision may be made with the Swann knife. The knife is directed carefully across the anterior chamber in the plane of the iris to engage Barkan's membrane or whatever abnormality that exists in front of the angle. It is important not to retract the knife prematurely, for this will cause the anterior chamber to become shallow and make the continuation of the operation impossible.

With the Barkan technique the surgeon positions the knife at about the junction of the upper and middle third of the trabecular area, and the assistant rotates the globe first in one direction, then in the other, sweeping approximately 120° of the angle. The knife is then withdrawn and the incision closed.

The patient is then positioned postoperatively on the side opposite the goniotomy site. The pupil is kept mobile.

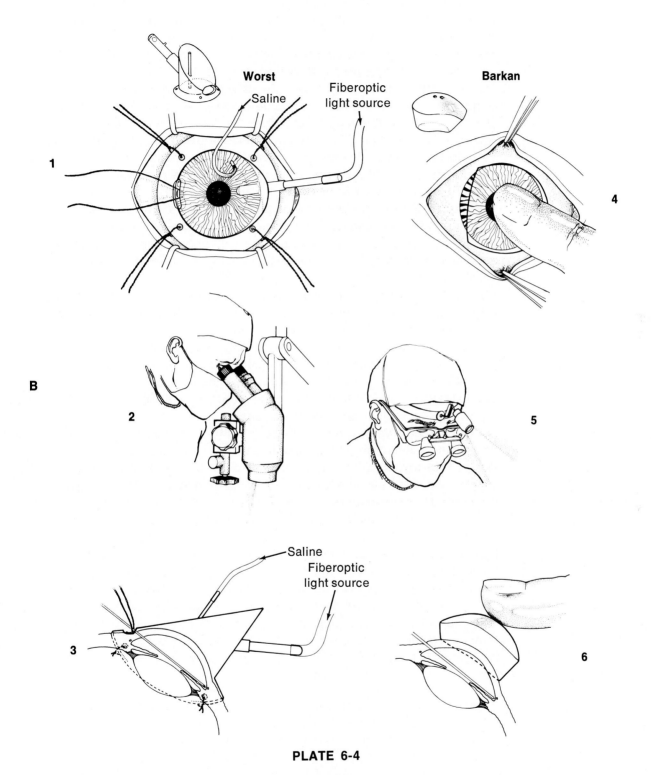

Worst

Saline

Fiberoptic
light source

1

Barkan

4

B

2

5

Saline
Fiberoptic
light source

3

6

PLATE 6-4

139

PLATE 6-5

A (1) The fenestrated Worst goniotomy knife has traversed the anterior chamber and engages the most superficial angle tissues lying above the plane of the iris at about the junction of the upper and middle thirds of the trabeculum.

(2) The Barkan knife has traversed the anterior chamber and engages the most superficial angle fibers above the plane of the iris.

B (1) While the operator stabilizes the Worst goniotomy lens with one hand, the other hand guides the goniotomy knife in a counterclockwise position, severing the superficial tissues. As the knife sweeps the angle, the iris may be seen to fall away and the angle deepens. This part of the goniotomy should be, in essence, a visual experience rather than a tactile experience. There should be no gritty feeling while the knife moves. If the surgeon notes any shallowing of the anterior chamber, he may ask the assistant to apply gentle pressure on the syringe that supplies saline solution through the fenestrated knife. During this procedure, however, it is important to avoid excess pressure on the plunger, as this will cause instantaneous clouding of the already compromised cornea and loss of the view of the chamber angle.

(2) The Barkan knife moves slightly counterclockwise while the assistant rotates the eye in a clockwise direction. This causes the angle more or less to sweep by the knife. Since the goniotomy knife is tapered, it will maintain a tight fit with the corneal incision only as long as it remains at its maximum distance in the anterior chamber. If the knife is retracted inadvertently, the anterior chamber will become shallow, and it will be necessary to remove the knife before completing the procedure if it appears that there is danger that the lens will be damaged.

C (1) The surgeon then sweeps the Worst knife in a clockwise direction, completing a goniotomy for approximately 3 to 4 clock hours.

(2) The Barkan knife shifts slightly in the clockwise direction while the assistant rotates the eye in a counterclockwise direction, achieving a goniotomy for 3 to 4 clock hours.

D At the conclusion of the procedure, the goniotomy knife is withdrawn from the anterior chamber with care taken to avoid traumatizing the iris or the lens. In nearly every case where a goniotomy has been performed properly, hemorrhage will occur in the angle at the site of the goniotomy. This should be irrigated gently with balanced salt solution. This minimal hemorrhage usually stops within 30 seconds to 1 minute. The corneal incision is closed with an 8-0 collagen suture. Balanced salt solution is used to reform the chamber. Postoperatively the infant is positioned to sleep on the side opposite the angle that received the goniotomy. This keeps blood and fibrin from collecting in the operated angle.

Goniotomy may be repeated in each eye three times if necessary. The first point of goniotomy should be the nasal angle. It is somewhat easier to perform a goniotomy in this position. The second goniotomy is done in the temporal angle. It is a bit more difficult to perform the procedure bringing the goniotomy knife over the patient's nose. The third goniotomy is positioned according to gonioscopy findings preoperatively.

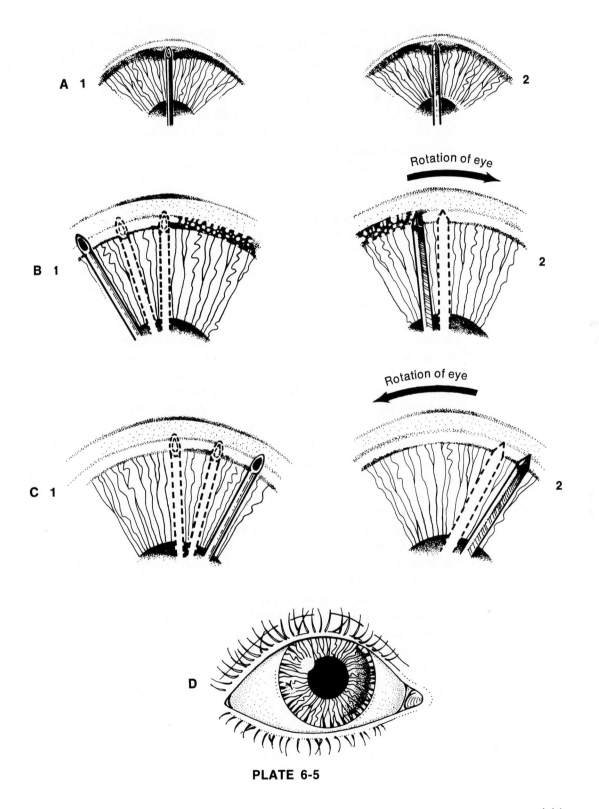

Rotation of eye

Rotation of eye

PLATE 6-5

Trabeculotomy

In cases of congenital glaucoma where extreme corneal haze makes it impossible to view the angle with a gonioprism, thereby making it impossible to perform a goniotomy in the usual way, trabeculotomy may be done. This procedure, when done successfully, should accomplish a "deep" goniotomy in which Schlemm's canal is opened into the anterior chamber directly in the operated area. This procedure is more difficult to control, we think, than a goniotomy, because of the uncertainty that accompanies localization and cannulation of Schlemm's canal from an external incision. This procedure, although theoretically sound, has not gained widespread acceptance. However, some surgeons prefer to use it even in instances where the cornea is clear.

PLATE 6-6

A After a small, limbus-based conjunctiva-Tenon's flap at the 12 o'clock position is prepared, a 5-mm incision is made in sclera at right angles to a tangent at the 12 o'clock position. A scratch incision is carried out with a No. 64 Beaver blade with careful inspection at each side of the incision to observe Schlemm's canal. When Schlemm's canal is transected, it is sometimes possible to observe a drop of clear fluid exuding from the cut ends. With Schlemm's canal identified, a 5-0 nylon suture is grasped in a needle holder and the suture is threaded into Schlemm's canal. This is a rather delicate and somewhat difficult maneuver, which is certainly much easier to describe than to perform. When the suture has been placed in Schlemm's canal and has passed without obstruction, the surgeon may be confident that the trabeculotomy instrument can be inserted in a similar fashion. A double-pronged trabeculotomy instrument is available in a right-hand and a left-hand model. The second prong offers a reference plane, assisting the surgeon in maintaining the trabeculotomy arm in a position parallel to the plane of the iris. Schlemm's canal also can be identified by making a deep trabeculectomy flap and unroofing a segment of the canal.

B The surgeon carefully threads the lower arm of the trabeculotomy instrument into Schlemm's canal on one side.

C When the trabeculotomy instrument has been properly placed, it is rotated, fracturing Schlemm's canal into the anterior chamber. The lower arm of the instrument is seen in the anterior chamber. When this is accomplished, the instrument is removed.

D The left-handed trabeculotomy instrument may then be introduced into the other opening into Schlemm's canal and the steps repeated.

E The incision is closed with an 8-0 collagen suture. The conjunctiva need not be closed.

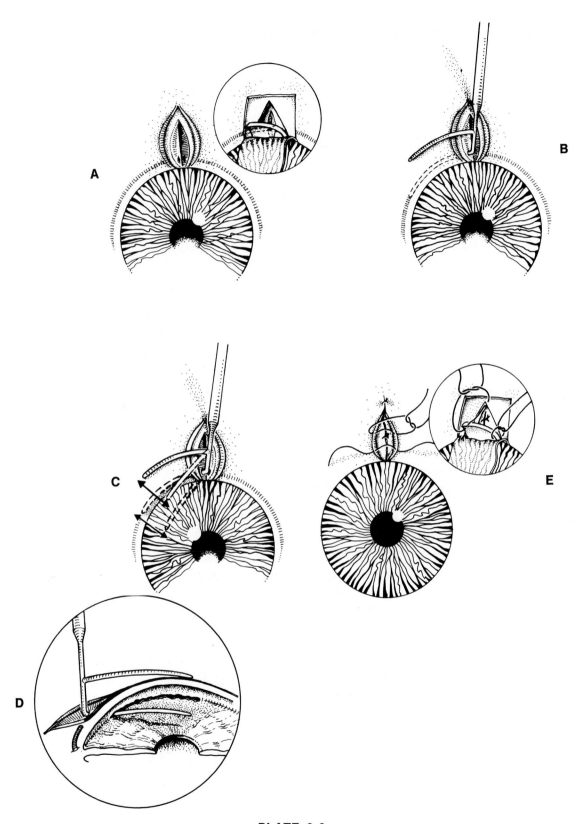

PLATE 6-6

143

The Scheie procedure (thermal sclerostomy)

In congenital glaucoma cases where goniotomy has failed after a reasonable number of times (usually three), a filtering procedure may be done. One preferred filtering procedure is the Scheie thermal sclerostomy. This procedure is also useful in cases of acquired glaucoma where medical treatment has been unsuccessful. The essence of the Scheie filtering procedure is a joining of the anterior chamber to sub-Tenon's space, allowing free access of anterior chamber contents to sub-Tenon's space. Since the pressure in the anterior chamber in glaucoma patients is higher than the pressure under conjunctiva-Tenon's flap, provided it remains open, the lowering of anterior chamber pressure is effected with drainage of aqueous out of the anterior chamber through the fistula site. Because of exuberant Tenon's capsule in children, filtering procedures are said to work less well in children than in adults.

PLATE 6-7

A The eye is rotated downward and an incision is made through conjunctiva and anterior Tenon's capsule approximately 10 mm posterior to the limbus and nasal to the superior rectus muscle. An incision is placed here to allow maximum protection for the bleb postoperatively. Also, if a second procedure must be done, the superior temporal quadrant can be employed. Care must be taken when rotating the eye downward to avoid lacerating conjunctiva and Tenon's capsule near the limbus. A large flap of conjunctiva and anterior Tenon's capsule is reflected down to the limbus. It is important to carry the flap over the peripheral cornea, exposing the surgical limbus and the anterior chamber angle beneath so that the incision may be made well anterior to the root of the iris and the ciliary body.

B A No. 64 Beaver blade is employed to make a scratch incision just on the corneal side of the limbal sulcus. This incision should be approximately 4 mm long.

C A 0.1- or 0.2-mm deep scratch is followed by a hot cautery. We use the single-battery, disposable cautery. The scratching and cautery are carried out for three to five alternate maneuvers until the anterior chamber is entered. This may be done either with the cautery or with the blade. The entry into the anterior chamber should be approximately 1 to 1.5 mm, and both sides of the incision should be adequately seared.

D Gentle pressure is applied on the cornea or to the posterior lip of the wound with a spatula, causing the iris to prolapse in the wound. If the iris does not prolapse spontaneously, it may be grasped with a fine forcep. Great care must be exercised to avoid traumatizing the lens.

E A small peripheral iridectomy is made.

F The anterior chamber is re-formed with balanced saline solution, and an 8-0 braided Vicryl suture is used to close the conjunctiva. The sutures may be running or interrupted. Care is taken to effect a watertight closure.

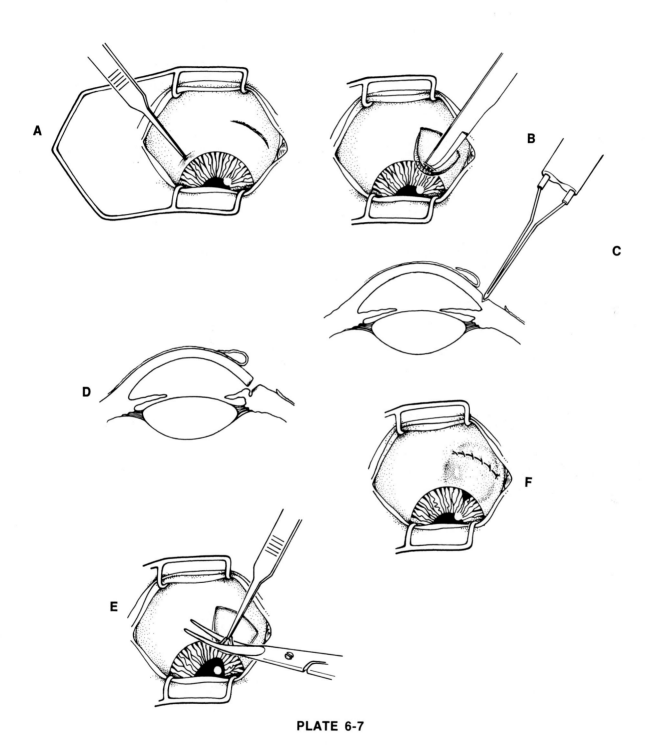

PLATE 6-7

145

Trabeculectomy

As an alternate filtering procedure to the Scheie thermal sclerostomy, trabeculectomy has been recommended. This procedure provides the advantage of the decreased likelihood of a prolonged flat chamber postoperatively, and the filtration rate can be controlled to a greater degree by alteration of the size and location of the scleral flap. There is not uniform agreement with regard to the comparative attributes of thermal sclerostomy and trabeculectomy. Either procedure may be employed if an external filtering procedure is indicated.

PLATE 6-8

A A conjunctival Tenon's flap, limbal based, is reflected over the cornea. A triangular incision is made and a scleral flap is undermined with the base at the limbus. The scleral flap is carried over the surgical limbus into the cornea.

B The flap should extend over the cornea so that in its most corneal extent it is anterior to the filtration angle.

C The triangular flap of sclera is reflected on over the cornea.

D This exposes the filtration angle beneath.

E The filtration angle is excised, and a peripheral iridectomy is performed. The excised portion of chamber angle should be 3 to 4 mm long and approximately 2 mm wide.

F The scleral flap is closed with one 7-0 or 8-0 absorbable synthetic suture at the apex of the triangle, and the conjunctiva is closed with a running suture of 7-0 absorbable synthetic suture.

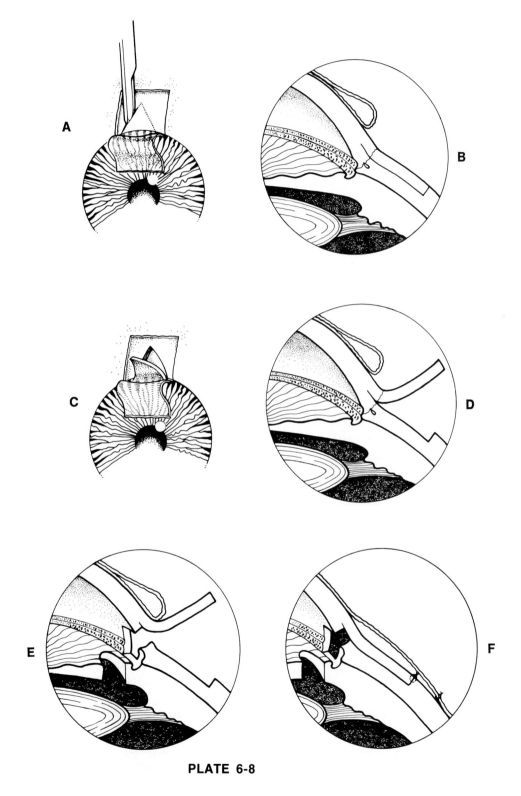

PLATE 6-8

147

Medical treatment

The medical treatment of both congenital and acquired childhood glaucoma is less successful than it is in adults. Congenital glaucoma caused by filtration angle abnormalities should be treated by a goniotomy when possible and by filtering procedures when goniotomy fails. Medical treatment is used only after failure of surgical treatment. In some cases of failed surgical and medical treatment, partial destruction of the ciliary processes and, therefore, reduction of aqueous output is accomplished by cyclocryotherapy. Some types of glaucoma that are present from birth or that originate in childhood as a result of a congenital abnormality are not amenable to goniotomy or filtering procedures. In most instances these patients are treated best by medical treatment, which may also be employed in other patients as a temporary measure before surgery.

Medical regimens for childhood glaucoma follow.

Miotics

Pilocarpine 1% to 4% may be used as often as one drop every 6 to 8 hours. Phospholine iodide 0.06% to 0.25% may be used once or twice a day.

Sympathetic agents

Epinephrine 1% may be used once or twice a day.

Beta adrenergic blocker

Timolol 0.25% to 0.5% may be used once or twice a day.

Carbonic anhydrase inhibitor

Diamox up to 10 mg/kg of body weight per day may be taken. Children do not ordinarily experience significant side effects from the medical treatment for glaucoma, with the exception of Diamox. When Diamox is taken, ample amounts of potassium should be ingested. This can be accomplished safely by eating fresh fruits, such as bananas and oranges, daily.

Cyclocryothermy

There are cases where medical treatment is not effective in controlling pressure, and pain is experienced or function is presumed lost, as measured by decrease in visual field in an older child or more commonly manifested as an increase in nerve head cupping. When surgery in the form of goniotomy or filtering procedures has failed or is not feasible, cryotherapy may be done. Using a probe that cools to −69° C, freezing spots are placed in a contiguous fashion around 270°. The freezing spots are made 4 mm from the limbus so that the freeze occurs over the ciliary body, engulfing it. Cyclocryotherapy must be done with general or dissociative anesthesia in a child. Postoperative pain and discomfort are reduced if 1.5 ml of 0.75% bupivacaine (Marcaine) is injected into the retrobulbar space. Cyclocryotherapy is ordinarily a last resort pressure control attempt in children who have useful vision. In eyes that are blind and painful but are not enucleated for various reasons, cyclocryothermy can be a very successful method of controlling pressure and pain.

148

PLATE 6-9

A The patient is taken to the operating room, and a general anesthetic is administered. This may be in the form of intubation inhalation agents, or ketamine may be used. One and one-half milliliters of 0.75% bupivacaine is injected into the retrobulbar area. A freezing probe is held on the conjunctiva 4 mm posterior to the limbus, just nasal to the superior rectus muscle insertion. The freeze is applied for 1 minute. The freezing is discontinued, and when the cryoadhesion to the conjunctiva has ceased, the probe is removed from the conjunctiva. This is continued two freezes to a quadrant for two to four quadrants. Each spot is ordinarily frozen twice.

B The freeze occurs in a more or less circular configuration, engulfing the ciliary processes, and destroying the ciliary epithelium, thereby reducing outflow.

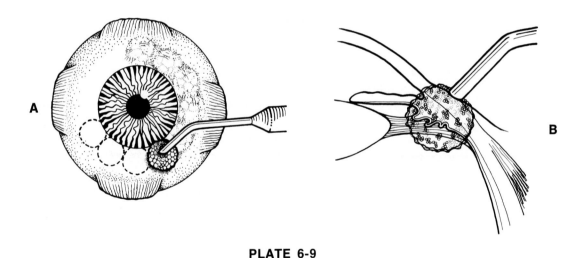

PLATE 6-9

149

OTHER FORMS OF GLAUCOMA

In addition to primary congenital (infantile) glaucoma, several other glaucomas of congenital origin occur in childhood. These have been classified by Shaffer and Hoskins[41] according to the tissues or structures involved.

Mesodermal
  Axenfeld syndrome (familial hypoplasia of the iris)
  Rieger syndrome
  Peters anomaly
  Marfan syndrome (systemic)
  Weill-Marchesani syndrome (systemic)
Ectodermal
  Aniridia
Trabecular dysgenesis
  Congenital (infantile) glaucoma
  Sturge-Weber syndrome
  Rubella
  Lowe syndrome
  Neurofibromatosis
  Rubinstein-Taybi syndrome

Axenfeld syndrome is characterized by a prominent Schwalbe line (posterior embryotoxon) with dense bands of iris tissue attached. The glaucoma that occurs develops between ages 5 and 25 years and behaves as open-angle glaucoma. It is inherited as an autosomal dominant trait. Medical treatment is preferred, but a filtering procedure is employed when medical management is no longer effective.

Rieger syndrome is characterized by hypoplasia of the iris stroma. When bands of iris tissue attach to the posterior cornea, the intraocular pressure becomes elevated. The condition is transmitted as an autosomal dominant trait. Glaucoma develops between ages 5 and 25 years. The treatment of glaucoma with Rieger syndrome is the same as for open-angle glaucoma: medical treatment first, and a filtering procedure if medical treatment fails.

Peters anomaly is similar to Rieger syndrome but includes central iridocorneal adhesions with corneal opacity. Successful corneal grafts have been done in young children with this condition.

Marfan syndrome consists of arachnodactyly, cardiac anomalies, subluxated lenses, and sometimes glaucoma that behaves in a manner similar to open-angle glaucoma.

Aniridia is a severe bilateral congenital ocular abnormality characterized by the complete or nearly complete absence of the iris. It occurs either sporadically or as a dominantly inherited characteristic with fairly complete penetrance. About 20% to 30% of patients with sporadic congenital aniridia have Wilms tumor. Conversely, the prevalence of aniridia in patients with Wilms tumor is approximately 1 in 73. Patients with aniridia have decreased visual acuity, but this ranges in certain pedigrees from 20/30 to 20/200 or worse. They frequently develop cataracts and almost always have a corneal pannus. Glaucoma occurs frequently, with the onset in the late preteens or early teens. This glaucoma is extremely difficult to treat medically or surgically. Grant and Walton have suggested prophylactic goniotomy in patients with aniridia, but final results with this treatment are not yet available. It has been suggested that anterior synechiae formed by a remnant of the iris in the aniridic patient eventually will obstruct the trabecular meshwork. The prophylactic goniotomy is aimed at preventing this occurence. The treatment of aniridia and its associated ocular abnormalities is a most discouraging aspect of pediatric ophthalmology. We have used pinhole lenses in these patients in an attempt to decrease nystagmus and enhance the development of vision. Results are inconclusive, although nystagmus has decreased in some patients. The presence of the vascular pannus with the contact lens creates a severe management problem. The glaucoma associated with aniridia is treated medically, and if this fails, it is treated with a filtering procedure or cyclocryotherapy.

In general, *congenital (infantile) glaucoma* bears little resemblance to its adult counterpart. It occurs much less commonly and when it does, the treatment modalities are ordinarily more complicated and less effective. The one exception with regard to treatment is primary congenital glaucoma. In this condition, a well-done goniotomy is effective in controlling pressure, but in a high percentage of patients visual acuity is poor (in the neighborhood of 20/100 or 20/200). The reason for this is that these eyes experience severe anatomical changes. They have corneal enlargement, tears in Descemet's membrane, and myopic astigmatism. When it occurs unilaterally, the amblyopiagenic factors of the anisometropia are considerable. Once glaucoma has been diagnosed in an infant or child, the patient must be followed carefully for the remainder of his or her life. Even after many years of controlled pressure, serious glaucoma can recur.

Sturge-Weber syndrome is a cutaneous hemangiomatosis that involves the area of distribution of the fifth cranial nerve. It is usually unilateral. The glaucoma occurs as a result of vascular abnormalities in the iris in the area of the filtration angle. It is treated in a manner similar to that for primary open-angle glaucoma. If surgery is required, a filtering procedure or cyclocryotherapy is done.

Maternal rubella causes significant damage to the ocular development of the fetus. Uveitis, glaucoma, and microphthalmos can result. The glaucoma is treated medically or surgically with a filtering procedure.

Lowe syndrome is rare and genetically determined. This is probably sex-linked in that it occurs predominantly in males. It is associated with bilateral cataracts and bilateral glaucoma. These conditions may be treated with goniotomy and lens removal. We did these procedures at the same time in one patient with success.

Patients with *neurofibromatosis* may develop plexiform neuromas in the area of the angle. They lead to increased intraocular pressure, which must be treated medically or by a filtering procedure.

Intraocular tumors that cause forward displacement of the lens and closure of the angle can result in acute glaucoma. We have seen this in one case of retinoblastoma and in several patients with retrolental fibroplasia. Glaucoma is

151

also said to occur in certain cases of persistent hyperplastic primary vitreous where traction causes forward displacement of the lens-iris diaphragm. The glaucoma asssociated with these diseases is treated by carrying out the proper treatment for the underlying disease.

Eyes that are traumatized in childhood are also prone to glaucoma. Blunt trauma that causes contusion and angle recession may be associated with a late-occurring glaucoma. Yanoff[*] has suggested that this type of glaucoma in angle recession is caused not by the actual physical disinsertion of the ciliary body, but by an endothelial cell growth curving in a sheet form extending over the filtration angle and the anterior surface of the iris. The angle recession merely is an indication that the eye has received severe trauma that could give rise to this overgrowth of endothelial cells. This type of glaucoma is treated medically or with a filtering procedure.

Postoperative glaucoma

Patients who have had surgery for congenital cataracts and who have had secondary membranes and discissions may develop glaucoma. These types of mechanical glaucoma, which probably arise from destruction of integrity of the filtration angle during the inflammatory process associated with the surgery or from peripheral anterior synechiae, can be difficult to treat. Medical treatment and cyclocryotherapy are the treatments of choice.

A long list of congenital ocular diseases has been associated with increased intraocular pressure. These glaucomas should be treated on an individual basis. When the eye is salvageable, every effort should be made to keep the pressure in a physiologic range, which could be considered in the low 20s to teens. If vision is not salvageable in this type of eye, the patient should be made comfortable if the eye is to be retained. This may be done by medical therapy (but usually not long-term Diamox) or by the use of cyclocryotherapy. In cases where an eye is blind, painful, and unsightly, enucleation is the treatment of choice. Filtering procedures are contraindicated in these eyes because of the risks of sympathetic ophthalmia.

Steroid-induced glaucoma

In the last several years, we have seen several cases of steroid-induced childhood glaucoma. Most of these have been the result of treatment of childhood ocular inflammatory conditions with topical steroids. Pressures in these cases have gone up into the high 20s and low 30s on topical steroid treatments that were required to control intraocular inflammation. Some of these patients have required topical glaucoma treatment along with their steroid treatment.

One patient we saw had used hydrocortisone ointment for 5 years. She began using the ointment after having it prescribed for an allergic conjunctivitis. She maintained the prescription on her own and took the medicine without supervision. When we saw her, her pressures were in the low 40s, the cup-disc ratio was 0.8, and visual fields were severely constricted.

----

[*]Yanoff, M.: Personal communication, 1978.

152

Chapter 7

BLEPHAROPTOSIS

BLEPHAROPTOSIS IN CHILDHOOD

Childhood blepharoptosis, regardless of the etiology, results in an objectionable appearance and is frequently associated with anisometropia, strabismus, and amblyopia. When the blepharoptosis is bilateral and severe, slowed motor development (such as delayed ambulation) can occur. The blepharoptosis itself and any of these associated findings represent a therapeutic challenge calling for individualized diagnosis and management. Knowledge of various surgical techniques and differential timing for surgical intervention is required. When a pediatric blepharoptosis patient is encountered, the very special requirements of that patient should be recognized, associated abnormalities evaluated, and appropriate treatment planned.

Evaluation

The initial evaluation of the blepharoptosis patient includes a thorough history and a general examination of the patient. A clear history of congenital blepharoptosis in the absence of both significant birth trauma and a history of familial or genetic disorders, combined with a negative general physical examination, leaves one with the isolated diagnosis of congenital blepharoptosis. Electron microscopy of the levator muscle and aponeurosis in such patients has consistently demonstrated dystrophic changes of these tissues. When the diagnosis is clearly that of congenital blepharoptosis without associated systemic abnormalities, one may proceed with evaluation of that patient, planning for the ultimate correction of the disorder. Although the visual axes may be occluded by the ptotic lids in the primary position, good vision may be preserved in downgaze. Congenital blepharoptosis, because of the shortened levator aponeurosis and muscle, always provides an unobstructed area for viewing in the lower fields. If the condition is bilateral, the child may adopt a head back, chin up position in order to better view his environment. It is rare for blepharoptosis alone to produce amblyopia. In virtually all cases where amblyopia has been demonstrated to be associated with blepharoptosis (a not infrequent finding), anisometropia and strabismus with amblyopia have been present. Whether the blepharoptosis is a contributing factor to the amblyopia under these circumstances remains unclear, as indeed does the issue of whether the blepharoptosis is in some way responsible for the development of these other factors. However, since most patients with unilateral blepharoptosis do not get amblyopia unless anisometropia is present, it is reasonable to assume that such amblyopia is at least one step removed from the blepharoptosis itself. Nevertheless, in the young child with severe bilateral blepharoptosis, an abnormal head position, and suspected delayed ambulation, a temporary or interim frontalis suspension procedure might be indicated until growth and development are such that a more permanent procedure can be undertaken. Unless such circumstances are present, it is generally better to delay surgical intervention until the preschool years for reasons that are discussed below. Thus, in the early evaluation of the child with blepharoptosis it is necessary to ascertain the presence or absence of associated abnormalities, both general and ocular. Surgery will seldom be done in the early months or years unless overriding factors described above are present.

In the older child who is being evaluated for the surgical correction of blepharoptosis, the relationship of the lid margin to the cornea and pupil should be charted with a simple line drawing. Photographs are desirable. A normal palpebral opening is about 9 mm in vertical dimensions. Symmetry should be present, with a variation of less than 0.5 mm between the two eyes. The upper lid margin ordinarily covers the upper limbus to a distance of 1 to 1.5 mm. The first step, therefore, is to sketch on the patient's chart the relationship of the lids to the globes. Notation is made as to the width of the palpebral fissure when the patient, with his head erect and without frontalis effort, is gazing levelly across the room.

154

Levator function is evaluated by asking the patient to look down at the floor. The examiner then holds the patient's head firmly against the head rest with the examiner's fingers and hand over the brow area so that frontalis effort is rendered ineffective. The patient is then asked to look at the ceiling. A comparison of the upper lid excursion between the two eyes is then measured. Normally the upper lid will elevate under such circumstances from 12 to 17 mm, and this elevation should be symmetrical. Children with congenital blepharoptosis will demonstrate a shortened upper lid on downgaze and reduced levator function on upgaze. This is due to the dystrophic changes in the levator aponeurosis and the levator muscle, which produce shortening as well as reduced function. If the blepharoptosis is of equal magnitude in upgaze and downgaze, a Mueller muscle weakness should be suspected. Under these circumstances the ptotic lid will elevate readily when 2½% phenylephrine (Neo-synephrine) drops are placed in the cul-de-sac. The amount of levator function along with the degree of ptosis determines the type of surgical procedure that will be performed as well as the amount of levator resection when that procedure is done. The patient is asked to chew and move his jaw from side to side to help determine the presence of Marcus-Gunn jaw winking syndrome.

Corneal sensation is evaluated, as is the presence of the Bell phenomenon. Corneal sensation is tested with a wisp of cotton drawn across the cornea. One measures the Bell phenomenon by attempting to force open the lids while the patient attempts to close the lids against the force of the examiner. Controversy has arisen regarding the value of an intact Bell phenomenon, since it has been demonstrated that the eye does not remain in elevation with prolonged lid closure or with sleep. We continue to note the presence of absence of this phenomenon, however, believing that early corneal drying or corneal irritation, even while sleeping, may initiate forced lid closure and elevation of the globe with a beneficial corneal wetting effect. Thus, the fact that the eye does not remain in elevation does not negate the value of voluntary lid closure and globe elevation. Most children can be cajoled into allowing both of these determinations. In those who cannot, the examination must be done while the child is restrained. Under these circumstances one can easily assess the presence or absence of an intact corneal sensation and at the same time observe the presence or absence of the Bell phenomenon.

With knowledge of (1) severity of the ptosis, (2) levator function, (3) mechanical and neural components, (4) corneal sensitivity, (5) the Bell phenomenon, and (6) the patient's age, motor development, and amblyopia potential, the type and timing of surgery can be planned.

Other factors that cause blepharoptosis must be recognized and recorded, such as mechanical problems from a hemangioma or von Recklinghausen disease, or neural causes, such as myasthena gravis or third nerve palsy. These should be recorded with photographs and drawings.

Mild to moderate unilateral or bilateral congenital blepharoptosis

Minor blepharoptosis that causes only cosmetic concern is not a significant factor until school age is approaching. At this time, peer pressure becomes a detrimental factor. For this reason, blepharoptosis that causes only a problem with appearance generally is treated only after the child reaches 4 or 5 years of age. The surgeon should plan to have all surgical correction completed before the significant social contact of the school years. Realistically, however, the timing of surgery is often modified by parental pressures. Earlier surgery can be done, but for reasons listed later in this chapter requires even greater concern on the part of the surgeon concerning the production of amblyopia as well as its prevention.

PLATE 7-1

A This patient demonstrates a mild unilateral blepharoptosis at age 3 years. Levator function is approximately 6 mm, compared with 15 mm on the normal side, and all other ocular and general physical aspects of this child are normal. In blepharoptosis such as this, the patient is examined at approximately yearly intervals and surgery is done at age 4 or 5 years. Our procedure of choice in this type of blepharoptosis is an external levator resection, roughly following Berke's table for the approximate amount of levator resected and for the lid position at the conclusion of surgery. In mild cases of blepharoptosis such as this, the lid is positioned at the point on the cornea where we want it to remain, after healing has taken place.

B This patient demonstrates a mild bilateral blepharoptosis with sparing of the visual axes and sufficient lid excursion to allow for vision without thrusting the head backward to a point where it will cause the child to topple backward. As with mild unilateral blepharoptosis, this patient (who is normal in all other respects from an ocular as well as general physical standpoint) will undergo bilateral external levator resection at age 4 or 5 years. Both lids will be elevated at the same procedure.

Insignificant degrees of unilateral and especially bilateral blepharoptosis may be left untreated if they do not produce a noticeable cosmetic deformity. Occasionally, such patients will seek relief as teenagers or adults either because of asymmetry of the lids or because of "bedroom eyes."

156

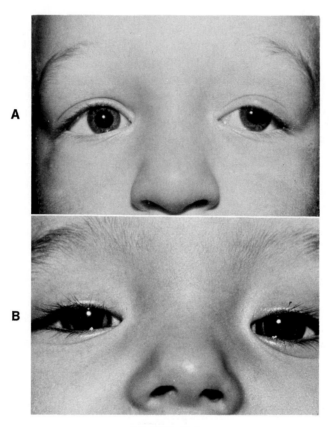

PLATE 7-1

157

Severe blepharoptosis

Retarded motor development can occur when both lids are ptotic to such an extent that the child must lean so far backward to clear the pupillary axis that balance is lost. In the crib, blepharoptosis is less of a problem because the child maintains a more or less supine position and is able to look downward to satisfy his visual needs without upsetting his posture. However, when attempts are made to sit up when the infant is between the ages of 5 and 7 months, the backward shift of the weight of the head caused by the uplifted chin may cause the child to topple over backward. This type of blepharoptosis may require treatment, usually to both lids during the rapid motor development years, up to the age of 1½. The procedure of choice is a frontalis suspension using a Prolene or Merseline suture or Prolene-reinforced bank sclera as sling material. Surgery is done on both lids at the same procedure. This procedure may be repeated if blepharoptosis recurs, using the same materials or irradiated, preserved fascia lata or autogenous fascia lata (the best material but not available in sufficient quantity until the child is older).

Significant unilateral congenital blepharoptosis that could cause amblyopia

Unilateral blepharoptosis that covers the pupillary axis can be a cause of amblyopia in an affected infant, but if so, is usually associated with anisometropia and strabismus. In such cases, we prefer to carry out blepharoptosis surgery when the patient is around 1 year of age. The aim of this surgery is to clear the pupillary axis when the child begins to sit up, not just to improve appearance. There should be no reason to be concerned about a 1-year-old infant's appearance from the standpoint of blepharoptosis. On the other hand, a functional loss of vision in one eye due to amblyopia must be avoided. This type of unilateral blepharoptosis is treated with a frontalis suspension. When a unilateral frontalis suspension is being considered for unilateral blepharoptosis, parents should be warned that there will be marked asymmetry of the palpebral fissures in downgaze. It is a good idea even to demonstrate this to the family by holding the patient's lid up while he looks down, or by showing them photographs. Bilateral suspension is advocated by some for this reason and because unilateral suspension results in less stimulus for frontalis usage.

PLATE 7-2

A Bilateral blepharoptosis that was managed in a unique way with the child holding one lid up to see while sitting up.

B Bilateral congenital blepharoptosis that hampered motor development, shown before and after bilateral frontalis suspension with a Prolene-reinforced scleral sling.

C Severe unilateral blepharoptosis, shown before and after treatment with a Prolene-reinforced scleral sling. This type of blepharoptosis can be associated with amblyopia.

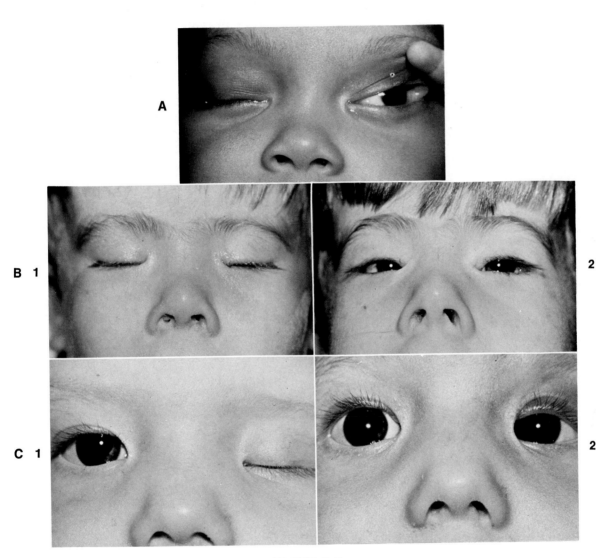

A

B 1   2

C 1   2

PLATE 7-2

SPECIAL TYPES OF BLEPHAROPTOSIS
Infantile Horner syndrome

Occasionally, a child will have mild blepharoptosis of one upper lid and pupillary miosis on the same side. This may be accompanied by heterochromia iridis with the lighter iris (more blue) on the involved side. Anhydrosis on the involved side and a history of birth trauma also may be noted. As with the previously mentioned types of blepharoptosis, a mild infantile Horner syndrome is not treated until later. If the blepharoptosis becomes a cosmetic problem, a tarsal conjunctival resection is an ideal procedure. It is important to point out to parents that the heterochromia iridis is an insignificant finding and that Horner syndrome is a nonprogressive, benign neurologic condition in this case. Its presence should be documented and confirmed early so that if noted later, extensive neurologic examinations are not undertaken. The blepharoptosis will be eliminated in a few seconds if phenylephrine is placed in the cul-de-sac. This is evidence of denervation hypersensitivity of the sympathetically innervated Mueller muscle.

PLATE 7-3

An 8-month-old infant demonstrating 2 mm of blepharoptosis of the right upper lid. He had a history of a difficult delivery. Note that the iris on the right is less pigmented and that the pupil is smaller.

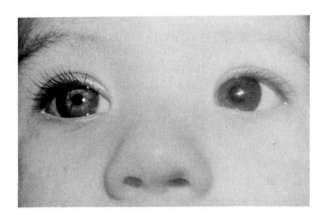

PLATE 7-3

Marcus Gunn jaw-winking phenomenon

The patient with Marcus Gunn jaw-winking phenomenon is an unusual type of patient who may have a mild to severe unilateral blepharoptosis in the primary position. However, during movement of the jaw away from the involved eye, the lid assumes a normal or sometimes excessively elevated position. The upper lid in these cases bounces up and down as the jaw moves. Diagnosis of this condition is relatively simple. If there is any suspicion, the patient is given candy or gum to chew. Chewing or voluntary movement of the jaw to the opposite side will, in nearly every case, bring out the typical lid movements because of the synkinesis between the motor nerve to the ipsilateral external pterygoid muscles and the levator muscle.

A useful rule of thumb for treatment of jaw winking follows.

1. If the ptosis is severe and the jaw winking relatively minimal, a frontalis suspension should be carried out.
2. If the jaw winking is severe with any degree of blepharoptosis, a levator extirpation should be done, followed by a frontalis suspension.
3. In certain cases where the blepharoptosis is moderate and the jaw winking is mild, an external levator resection may be carried out.

PLATE 7-4

This patient demonstrates the typical findings of Marcus Gunn jaw-winking phenomenon.

A With his jaw in the normal position a moderate ptosis of the left upper lid is present.

B When the jaw is moved, the lid elevates because of an aberrant connection between the motor root of the fifth and third nerves.

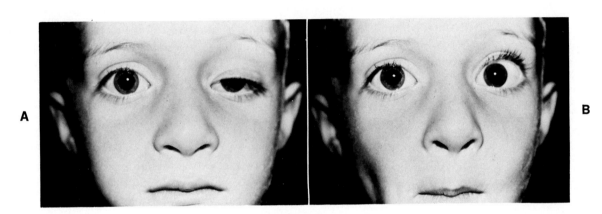

A

B

PLATE 7-4

Blepharoptosis with a prosthesis (PLATE 7-5, A)

Often after an enucleation and fitting of a prosthesis, blepharoptosis is present, which cannot be relieved entirely by prosthesis modification. This may be treated in a variety of ways. We have had most success with a tarsal conjunctival resection in very mild cases and a levator resection via the skin approach in the more severe cases.

Traumatic blepharoptosis (PLATE 7-5, B)

Traumatic blepharoptosis can occur after a variety of injuries to the upper lid. At least 1 year should pass before any surgical treatment is carried out in cases of blepharoptosis resulting from blunt trauma. When surgical treatment is indicated, it should be planned on the basis of levator function and the amount of blepharoptosis. Either a tarsal conjunctival resection (for mild blepharoptosis) or a levator resection or repair of an aponeurosis dehiscence (for more severe blepharoptosis) should be carried out. Lid lacerations causing blepharoptosis should be treated immediately by reattaching the severed aponeurosis. This patient demonstrates (1) severe posttraumatic blepharoptosis evident after the initial swelling has subsided and (2) partial recovery after 6 months.

Ptosis after a third nerve palsy (PLATE 7-5, C)

Some of the most difficult problems in ocular motility and blepharoptosis treatment occur after third nerve palsy, particularly when aberrant regeneration is present. If ptosis after third nerve palsy is severe in the primary position, a frontalis suspension may be carried out. If blepharoptosis is mild, a levator resection can be done. Unfortunately, in downgaze or in adduction, the blepharoptosis will disappear and actually give way to a widened palpebral fissure. Treatment in these cases can only be a compromise at best. These patients have a higher incidence of corneal exposure and drying postoperatively.

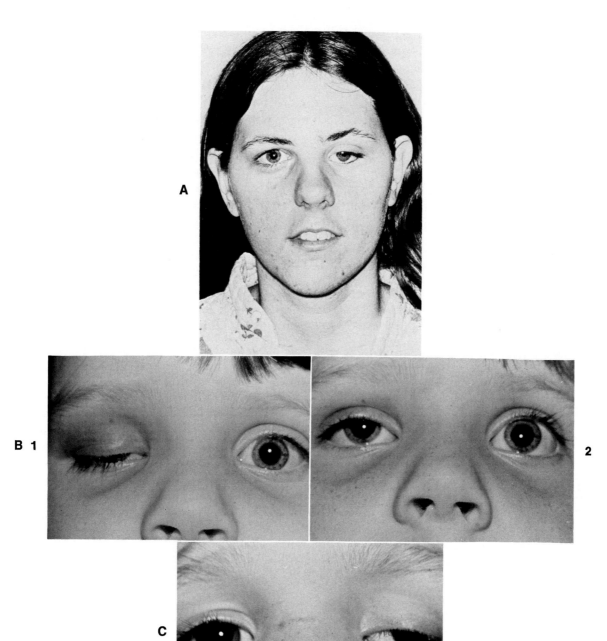

PLATE 7-5

165

Ptosis from mechanical causes

PLATE 7-6, A to C

A **(1)** A giant hairy nevus caused a remarkable blepharoptosis in this infant. A pediatrician attending this infant in the first week of life recognized the amblyopiagenic potential or this blepharoptosis. **(2)** The patient was referred, and subsequently the giant hairy nevus was removed when the patient was 6 weeks old, and a full-thickness skin graft was applied to the area. **(3)** The child has normal vision and an equal refractive error 4 years later. This case points out the importance of teamwork and an awareness of amblyopia on the part of physicians other than ophthalmologists.

B Hemangioma of the upper lid and adnexal area sometimes cannot be treated adequately. It will usually disappear or diminish in size through an involutional process, but large hemangiomas causing blockage of the pupil are accompanied by amblyopia. Occasionally, a smaller hemangioma may produce astigmatism and subsequent amblyopia. This type of lesion may require removal for cosmetic and functional reasons. **(1)** Before and **(2)** three weeks after 200 rads external beam irradiation.

C Von Recklinhausen disease with plexiform neuroma of the upper lid can cause a severe blepharoptosis. This is treated by partial excision of the neurofibroma and levator resection as needed, but this surgery can be difficult, and total removal of the neuroma is rarely possible.

Extraocular muscle fibrosis (PLATE 7-6, D)

Patients with extraocular muscle fibrosis present a typical picture of severe bilateral blepharoptosis and bilaterally hypodeviated eyes. On attempted elevation, there is a marked spasm of convergence with wrinkling of the brow, but very little elevation of the lids. These patients should be treated with appropriate extraocular muscle surgery on the medial and inferior rectus muscles at a young age. In many cases, the lids will follow the eyes into a more acceptable position. Brow suspension or levator resection may be done later if the lid position does not become satisfactory.

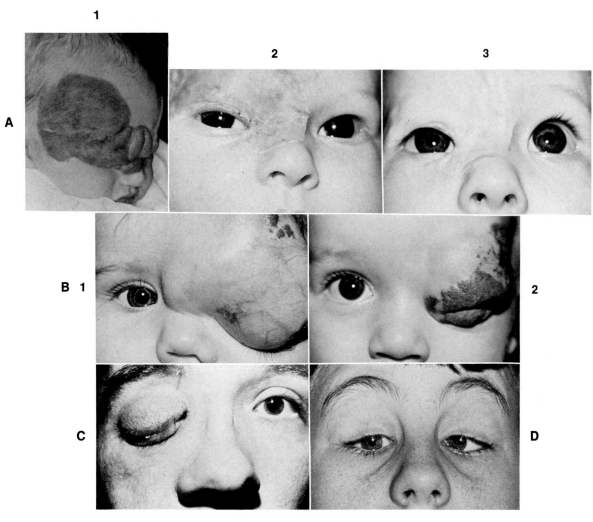

PLATE 7-6

Blepharophimosis syndrome

Blepharophimosis, blepharoptosis, epicanthus inversus, and telecanthus constitute a real therapeutic challenge. The condition usually is transmitted as an autosomal dominant trait but can occur sporadically. Affected children usually are of normal intelligence. The syndrome presents a fairly constant picture of little, if any, levator function. Either a levator resection or frontalis suspension is required to treat the blepharoptosis, and an epicanthus procedure is also indicated. Our choice is the Roveda procedure.

When 2 to 4 mm of levator function is present, a levator resection can be done, but because of a frequently abnormal anterior insertion of the septum orbitale, dissection is more difficult. However, when done carefully, the results can be gratifying. Whatever type of blepharoptosis procedure is done, both lids and both canthal areas are operated on at the same procedure.

In most cases of the blepharophimosis syndrome, frontalis slings are done bilaterally.

PLATE 7-7

This patient demonstrates bilateral blepharoptosis, epicanthus inversus, blepharophimosis, and telecanthus.

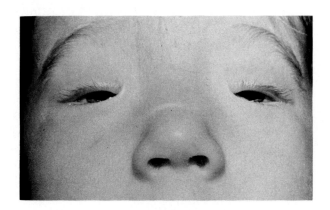

PLATE 7-7

TREATMENT OF BLEPHAROPTOSIS
Frontalis suspension

We have employed frontalis or brow suspension of the lid, using human, glycerin-preserved sclera since 1969. Because of early failures, presumably due to absorption of the implanted sclera, nonabsorbable suture, first 4-0 Supramid and then 5-0 Prolene, is now added to the sclera for a more permanent lid-lifting effect.

After removal from the glycerin-filled storage bottle, the scleral shell is placed in polymyxin (Neosporin) for 5 minutes, after which it is transferred to sterile saline solution for further rehydration.

PLATE 7-8

A The sclera is cut in the manner of a spiral similar to the technique one would use in peeling an apple. The strip of sclera so produced may be anywhere from 2 to 4 mm wide. One scleral shell will produce *two* 150-mm strips, each of which is adequate to suspend one eyelid.

B The 5-0 Prolene suture is woven through the scleral strip at approximately 5-mm intervals. When this is completed, the needles are cut from the ends of the Prolene suture.

C Two Stevens muscle hooks are useful in determining the inner extent of each lid incision. Ordinarily, the nasal lid incision is in line with the nasal limbus, and the temporal lid incision is made at the junction of the middle and temporal third of the cornea.

D After the two lid incision sites have been marked with a sterile pen about 2 mm above the lash line, a forehead mark is placed central to the lid marks. Two additional, symmetrical marks are then placed in the brow, completing the pentagon. A No. 15 Bard-Parker blade is used to make the incision through the skin and subcutaneous connective tissue. Each incision is less than 5 mm long.

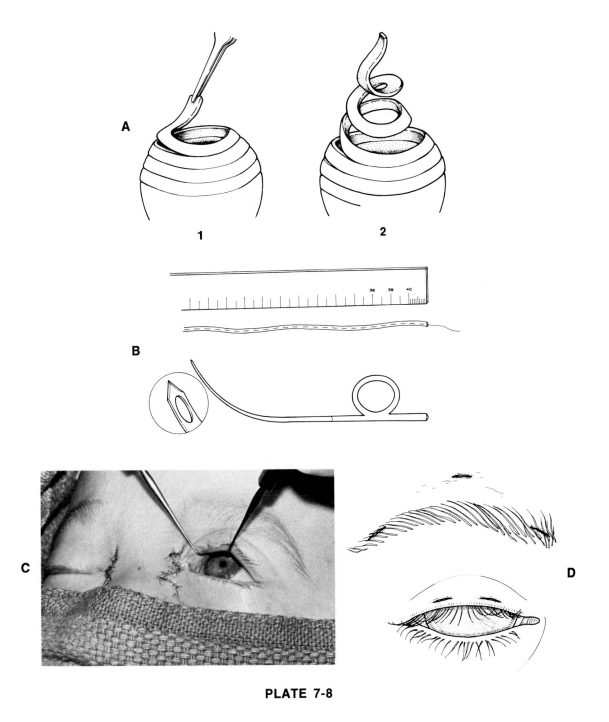

A

1   2

B

C

D

PLATE 7-8

171

PLATE 7-9

A A Wright needle is inserted into the nasal lid incision and passes out through the temporal lid incision. The eye of the Wright needle is loaded with the Prolene-reinforced scleral strip, and the needle is withdrawn through the subcutaneous tunnel in the lid.

B Each of the brow incisions is entered with the empty Wright needle; then the needle is loaded and withdrawn with the Prolene-reinforced scleral band.

C Finally, the Wright needle is inserted into the apical incision to the nasal and then the temporal side, withdrawing each end of the scleral band.

D The Prolene is then removed from the scleral strip to a point where the suture may be tied to itself. This produces an elevation of the lid to a point approximately at the upper limbus. The sclera is then pulled upward and sutured to itself with a buried 5-0 Merseline suture. The central and occasionally the brow incisions are closed with one or more 6-0 nylon or synthetic absorbable sutures. Special care should be taken to undermine skin superiorly at the apical incision so that there will be ample room to bury the knots. This incision may be the site of a pyogenic granuloma if suture ends are too superficial.

E A failed sling preoperative and postoperative redo of a bilateral Prolene-reinforced scleral frontalis sling.

Other materials are used for frontalis suspension, including autogenous fascia lata, irradiated cadaver fascia, and a variety of nonabsorbable sutures and plastic materials. If the child is old enough to have autogenous fascia lata available, this material should be considered, because its longevity is superior.

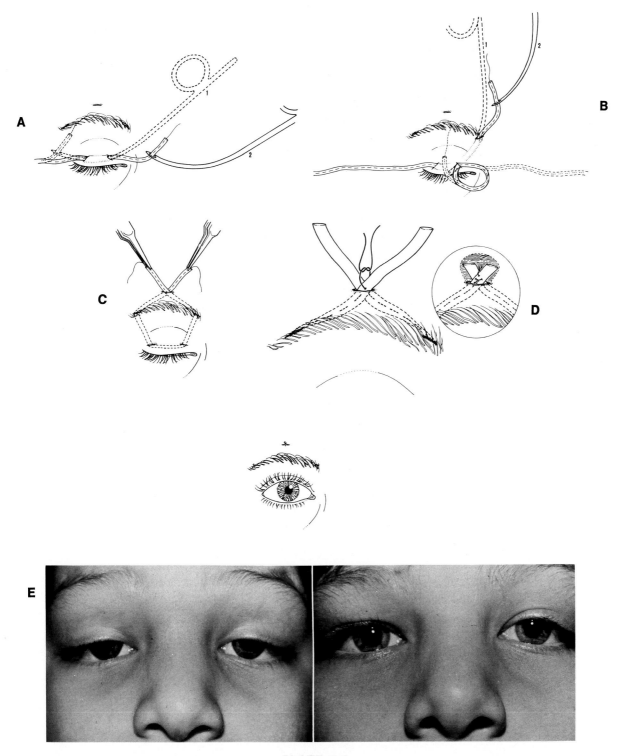

PLATE 7-9

External levator resection with conjunctival sparing

External levator resection with conjunctival sparing is an extremely useful modification of the Berke external levator resection. It requires a more meticulous dissection to free Mueller's muscle from underlying conjunctiva, but when performed properly, this procedure produces very rewarding results.

PLATE 7-10

A The procedure is begun by outlining the intended location for the lid fold on the operated eye. One-percent lidocaine with epinephrine 1:100,000 may be injected subcutaneously.

B An incision is made along the previously described line with a No. 15 Bard-Parker blade, penetrating skin and subcutaneous connective tissue. Scissors are used to separate the orbicularis muscle and expose the levator aponeurosis.

C Dissection is carried out between the orbicularis muscle and the levator aponeurosis over the tarsus to a point a few millimeters from the lid margin. Care should be taken to avoid damage to the lash bulbs. Dissection is continued upward preaponeurotically toward the orbital rim, identifying fat through the intact septum orbitale.

D The orbital septum may be **(1)** left intact or **(2)** severed here, depending on how much levator is to be resected.

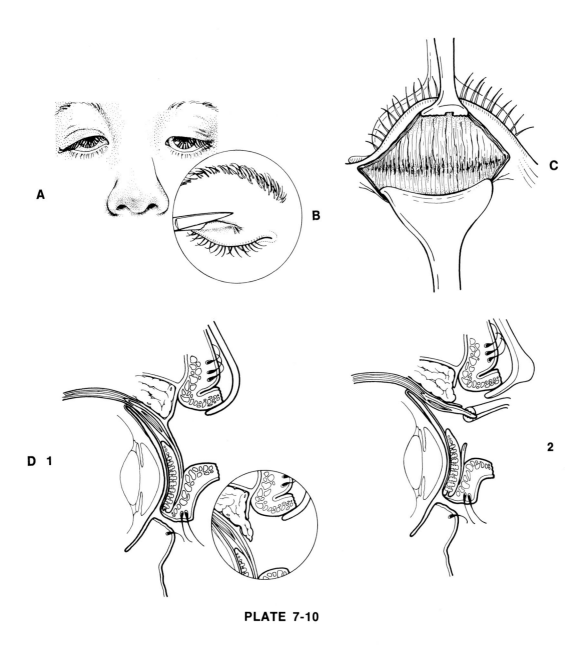

PLATE 7-10

175

PLATE 7-11

A The levator aponeurosis is then dissected free from the tarsus. This dissection may be difficult to initiate because of the very thin fusion of levator aponeurosis and tarsus.

B At the superior tarsal border, the plane between Mueller's muscle and conjunctiva is easier to develop. After the plane has been established, dissection is completed to the fornix with a dampened, cotton-tipped applicator. (The eye is shown without a corneal protector to emphasize the thinness of the conjunctiva.)

C The levator aponeurosis is placed in a blepharoptosis clamp, and the medial and lateral horns are cut. The degree to which the horns are severed depends on how much levator resection is required.

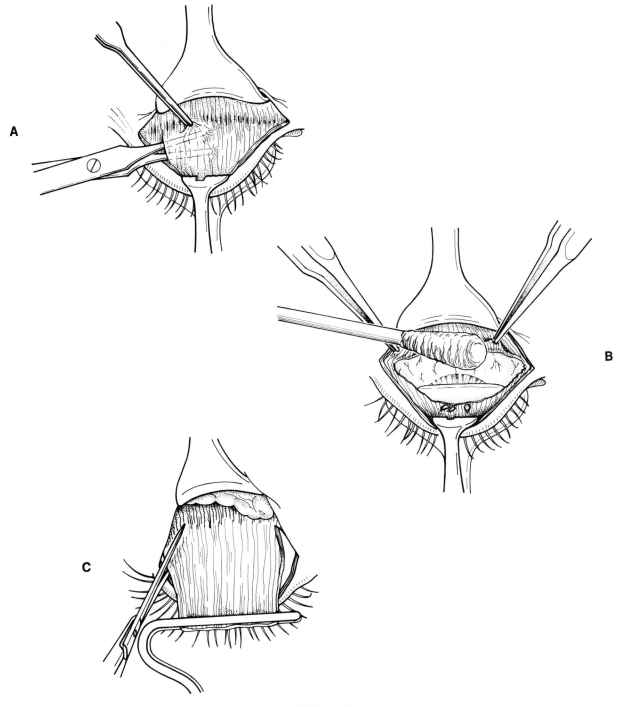

A

B

C

PLATE 7-11

PLATE 7-12

A Three 5-0 synthetic absorbable sutures are placed in the center, medial, and lateral aspects of the tarsus at its midpoint, and the double-armed sutures are brought up to the predetermined distance on the levator aponeurosis and are passed through the aponeurosis from below. It is always difficult to establish a formula for the correct amount of levator resection. It is axiomatic to say that the more severe the blepharoptosis, the more levator muscle must be resected. Berke's tables are generally reliable guides. As a rule of thumb, the smallest levator resection for congenital cases of a small amount of blepharoptosis with 8 to 10 mm of levator function should be in the neighborhood of 10 to 12 mm. In severe blepharoptosis of 5 mm or more, with 3 to 4 mm of levator function, 22 to 28 mm of levator resection may be carried out. Intermediate amounts of blepharoptosis and levator function are titrated accordingly.

B The sutures are tied over the levator aponeurosis after the appropriate amount of levator aponeurosis has been resected.

C It is now important to view the contour and height of the lid. If the contour is not satisfactory, it is adjusted by repositioning the sutures. After the final tie on the surface of the levator, the sutures are then brought out through the skin edges and retied. This produces a very satisfactory lid fold. Several interrupted sutures may be placed between these three anchoring sutures to close the lid. No dressing is used postoperatively. Plain 10% sulfa ointment without steroid is used postoperatively and is used two or more times a day for the next week. The family is given lubricating ointment for use as needed for the first few days.

D Preoperative and postoperative bilateral external levator resection.

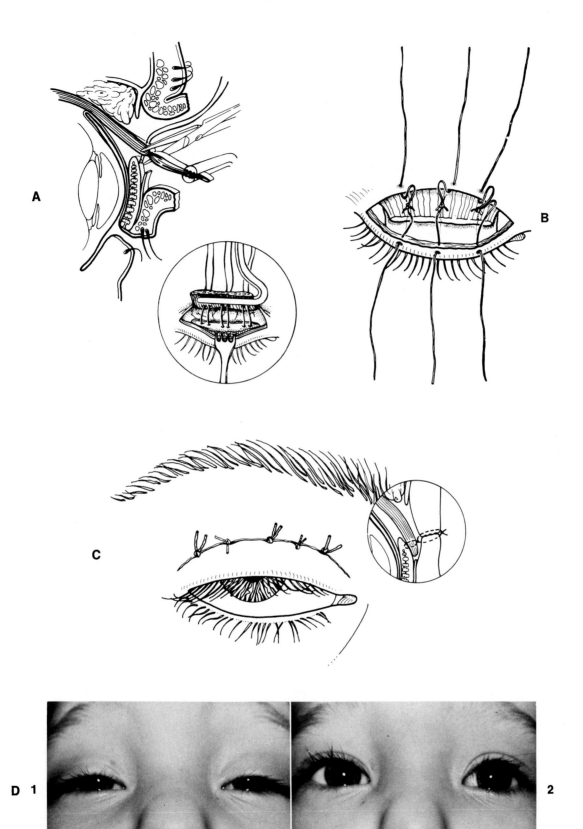

PLATE 7-12

Roveda procedure

PLATE 7-13

A The Roveda procedure is a modified Y-V plasty for treatment of an epicanthal fold.

B Two reference points are made, delineating the amount of nasalward shift desired for the medial canthus after the fold has been smoothed by nasalward traction. These points are connected with a line and labeled A and A'. Two lines are then drawn at an obtuse angle above and below the nasalmost extent of this line from point A. These lines are approximately the same length as the reference line. Two additional curvilinear lines are drawn from point A above and below at about 45°. These lines are also approximately the same length as the line A-A'.

C The four lateral triangular flaps are undermined, and point A is brought to point A', point B is brought to point B', and point C is brought to point C'. The excess skin flaps are excised, and the adjoining skin edges are sutured with either 6-0 nylon or 6-0 synthetic absorbable sutures. The latter causes some increased skin reaction, but it is very satisfactory in that it does not require removal.

D This patient demonstrates a preoperative and postoperative bilateral Roveda procedure and frontalis suspension of the upper lid.

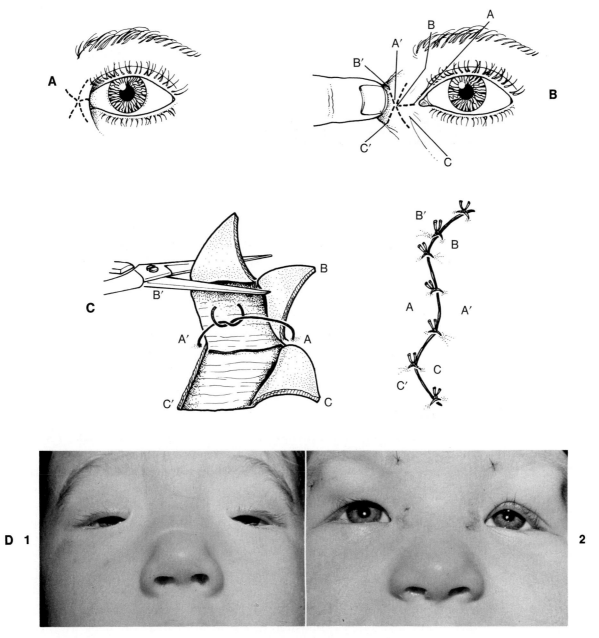

PLATE 7-13

Chapter 8

THE RETINA

Retinal diseases, including those of the vitreous and optic nerve, occurring in the pediatric age group differ from those occurring in adults, and examination and treatment techniques also differ a great deal. Both subjective and objective evaluation may be more difficult in the child because of the lack of cooperation in the young patient and also because of physical limitations, such as the presence of tunica vasculosa lentis in the premature infant. However, in spite of these difficulties, accurate diagnosis is possible, and effective treatment can be carried out as in the adult. As with other aspects of pediatric ophthalmology, the fact that the task may be difficult is no reason for not doing it. In some instances, it is necessary to use sedation or anesthesia to accomplish the required retinal examination.

EXAMINATION TECHNIQUES

Examinations of retinal *function* are subjective (visual acuity, color vision, visual fields, and so on) and objective (for example, electroretinogram [ERG], electrooculogram [EOG], and visually evoked response [VER]) (see Chapter 1). These tests may be carried out as indicated and when possible according to the level of cooperation in the individual patient.

The *appearance* of the retina, vitreous, and optic nerve can be evaluated utilizing one or more of the following techniques.

Direct ophthalmoscopy

Direct ophthalmoscopy can be difficult to accomplish in a young, awake, uncooperative child, but with patience on the part of the examiner, it can be done. Adequate pupillary dilatation is essential. When a satisfactory view can be obtained with the direct ophthalmoscope, the increased magnification obtained provides an excellent means of studying the disc, the macula, or a specific lesion of the posterior pole.

Indirect ophthalmoscopy

The ease with which the retina can be viewed with this technique makes indirect ophthalmoscopy the standard for pediatric retinal examination. The 30 D lens is used for scanning the retina. The 20 D lens is used for more detailed study of the disc and macula or specific lesions. A scleral depressor may be used for study of the peripheral retina, ora serrata, and pars plana. The use of a small lid speculum after a drop of topical anesthetic facilitates retinal examination in the premature or young infant.

Hruby lens

In a patient able to cooperate for examination at the slit lamp, the Hruby lens affords a detailed view of specific retinal areas in the posterior pole.

Goldmann lens

Peripheral lesions as well as posterior lesions and the anterior chamber angle can be studied with the Goldmann lens.

Retinal photography

Posterior pole and midperipheral lesions can be photographed using either a table-mounted or portable retinal camera.

Fluorescein angiography

The study of certain fundus lesions is enhanced by the use of fluorescein injected intravenously followed by fundus photography. This is particularly useful for early evaluation of the flecked retina syndrome.

A-scan ultrasonography

With opaque media, both the configuration and tissue characteristics of intraocular and intraorbital lesions can be studied in a child of any age with A-scan ultrasonography.

B-scan ultrasonography

A two-dimensional view of intraocular and intraorbital lesions can be obtained readily in a child of any age with B-scan ultrasonography.

DEVELOPMENTAL ABNORMALITIES
Coloboma

Failure of closure of the fetal fissure produces a coloboma of the retina and choroid. These defects occur sporadically and are bilateral in 60% of cases. The typical coloboma is located inferiorly and slightly nasally, although large colobomas can occupy the major portion of the inferior fundus. The coloboma bed consists of ectatic sclera with absent or abnormal choroidal and retinal vessels and a thin sheet of dysplastic retina. The choriocapillaris, Bruch's membrane, and pigment epithelium are absent in the area of the coloboma, and a visual field defect coincides with the coloboma. This condition may cause a severe visual defect if the macula or optic nerve is involved.

183

Optic nerve anomalies

Developmental anomalies of the optic nerve may be associated with central nervous system developmental defects, which may have local and systemic implications. Minor or major variations in optic nerve morphology do not indicate a need for further study, but a midfacial deformity or anomaly found in association with a developmental disc anomaly does warrant further investigation. It is not the type of optic nerve anomaly that indicates the presence of an associated central nervous system or cranial base deformity, but rather its association with midfacial defects.

Types of optic nerve anomalies seen in association with basal encephalocele are (1) disc pallor, (2) pits of the optic discs, (3) coloboma of the discs, (4) dysplasia, (5) megalopapilla, (6) situs inversus of the discs, (7) atypical coloboma, and (8) morning glory disc. The morning glory deformity consists of a deep excavation and enlargement of a pink nerve head with a whitish tissue, presumably glial, in its center. The disc is surrounded by an annulus of chorioretinal pigment disturbance. Blood vessels emerge radially from the periphery of this excavated disc, giving the appearance of a morning glory. When this or other types of optic nerve anomalies are found in a patient who has even a mild midfacial defect, x-ray films, including study of the base of the skull, should be carried out. Optic nerve anomalies may be seen in association with absent septum pellucidum, hypoplasia of the optic chiasm, tract, and pituitary gland with associated hormonal deficiencies. Bitemporal visual field defects may occur as a result of hypoplasia of the chiasm or as a result of compression of the chiasm when it is included in a basal encephalocele.

Hypoplasia of the optic nerve

A congenital decrease in or absence of nerve fibers emanating from the ganglion cell layer leads to hypoplasia of the optic nerve. This condition occurs sporadically and may be either unilateral or bilateral. An increased frequency in children of diabetic mothers has been reported. If few or no axon fibers are present, visual acuity is severely reduced. If adequate fibers are present, vision may be only minimally reduced. Clinically, hypoplasia of the optic nerve appears as a small nerve with normal-sized vessels. A "double ring" sign is formed by a scleral ring surrounding a smaller central nerve formed by glial elements that contain a reduced number of nerve fibers. A pigmented border surrounds these structures where the retinal pigment epithelium ends. When this condition occurs in one eye with some nerve fibers present, a functional amblyopia may be superimposed on an organic visual deficit; therefore, in some cases patching for amblyopia has been helpful. When hypoplasia occurs bilaterally, the septum pellucidum is frequently absent, porencephaly may occur, and involvement of the pituitary area in the hypoplastic process may lead to growth hormone deficiencies, usually manifest at age 3 or 4 years. Short stature and other endocrine defects may be present.

184

PLATE 8-1

A Morning glory disc.
B Atypical coloboma.
C Midline facial defect with blind sinus tract in the philtrum.
D Bony defect at the base of the skull.

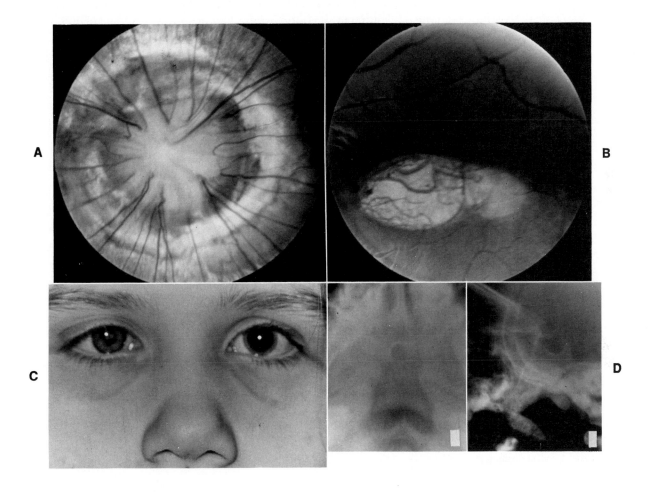

Congenital falciform folds

Congenital falciform folds of the retina emanate from the disc and usually course inferiorly and temporally to the retinal periphery, extending to the ciliary processes. The fold may be several millimeters high and associated with localized retinal detachment and macular degeneration. Visual acuity depends on the extent of macular involvement. Involvement may be bilateral or unilateral, and the condition, except for secondary retinal detachment (which occurs in some cases), is stable.

Congenital retinoschisis

This condition occurs in males, being transmitted as a sex-linked recessive disorder. The retina is split in the nerve fiber layer. These cystic changes may extend from the ora seratta to the optic nerve. The macula has typical changes that assume a spokelike configuration. When this macular appearance is seen in a young man, careful study of the peripheral retina should be undertaken. Vitreous membranes are seen in about one half the patients with retinoschisis. Secondary retinal detachment may occur if a hole develops in the outer retinal layer. Treatment of the schisis per se is not effective. We have seen attempts at delineating the area of schisis with photocoagulation fail in two patients. Older patients should be followed for progression with retinal photographs and visual field determination. Absolute scotomas are present in the visual fields corresponding to the affected retinal areas.

Persistent hyperplastic primary vitreous

A persistence of the hyaloid vessels connecting the disc and posterior lens leads to a significant ocular anomaly. The condition is unilateral, affects males and females equally, and invariably occurs in a small eye. The corneal diameter is reduced by 0.5 mm to 2.5 mm. The retrolental involvement of persistent hyperplastic primary vitreous (PHPV) is the most troublesome to the eye. A plaque may form on the posterior lens capsule with a fibrous mesh extending to the ciliary processes, which are elongated. Contraction or fracture of this fibrous area can cause sudden rupture of the lens capsule with abrupt maturation of a cataract. Milder forms of PHPV occur with only a thin strand of tissue connecting the disc and lens and with little or no ciliary process involvement. These eyes may remain healthier if the cataract and anterior hyaloid stalk are removed, but visual rehabilitation (other than the restoration of the peripheral field) of these eyes is not likely to be successful.

PLATE 8-2

A Hypoplasia of the optic nerve.
B Spokelike macular changes in retinoschisis.
C Persistent hyperplastic primary vitreous.

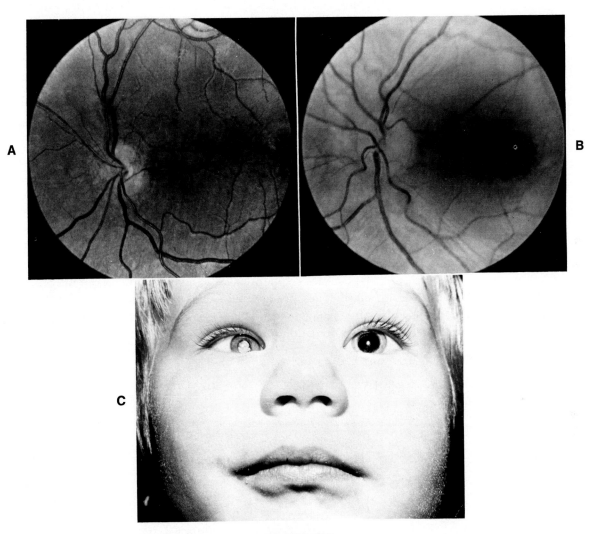

PLATE 8-2

187

Medullated nerve fibers

Normally, medullation of the axons of the ganglion cell layer stops at the lamina cribrosa, but in about 0.5% of people (usually males) medullation of the nerve fiber layer of the retina produces a featherlike, whitish growth usually extending for a few disc diameters above and below the disc, although isolated peripheral islands of medullation may appear. Except for a variable scotoma in the area of the medullated fibers, vision is not affected. The condition is stable and represents more of a curiosity than a significant pathologic condition, although in some cases, high myopia of the involved eye is present, particularly when the medullation is heavy.

Myopia

Severe, progressive, or high myopia is generally inherited as an autosomal recessive disorder, whereas milder degrees of myopia may be dominantly inherited but usually are not considered diseases. The severely myopic eye is characterized by steeper corneal meridia, by increased spherical shape of the lens, by increased anterior-posterior globe diameter, or by a combination of these findings. Pathologic changes in high myopia are generally confined to the enlargement and distortion of the posterior globe. The fundus changes of high myopia (−6.00 D or more) include thinning of the retinal layers, which gives the fundus a blond appearance. The retinal lamellae may be separated from the temporal side of the optic nerves, producing a pigmented temporal crescent. Peripherally, retinal degenerative changes including tears and holes are found frequently. Retinal detachment often occurs, particularly after mild trauma. The entire posterior segment usually develops a posterior bulge, creating a posterior staphyloma; or cracks in Bruch's membrane (lacquer cracks) appear. Macular hemorrhage and pigment changes (Fuchs spots) with disciform macular changes are frequent and cause significant reduction in vision.

PLATE 8-3

A Medullated nerve fibers.
B Myopia.

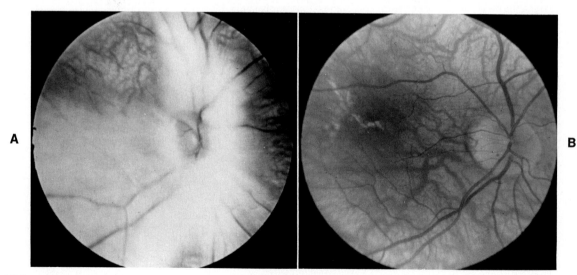

A

B

PLATE 8-3

RETINOPATHY OF PREMATURITY (ROP)
History

Retinopathy of prematurity (ROP), or retrolental fibroplasia (RLF), has been defined as a pathologic fibrous process involving the retina. First recognized as a disease entity by Terry[44] in 1942, the disorder was determined a decade later to be related to oxygen administration in the neonatal period of a premature infant. With the implication of oxygen in the pathophysiology of the disorder, oxygen use was curtailed, first in the United Kingdom and later in the United States. A definite increase in infant mortality and cerebral palsy occurred in each country as oxygen usage was decreased.

Animal studies and clinical information have served to further elucidate the pathophysiology of this potentially blinding disorder. The relative maturity or immaturity of the incompletely developed retinal blood vessels is the key to the determination of susceptibility to RLF. That is, acute changes of RLF have been produced in laboratory animals under a variety of conditions and with varying oxygen loads, but cicatricial RLF has yet to be produced in an animal model or in a mature retina, either in the laboratory or in human beings. Mature retinal vasculature is not susceptible to adverse effects of oxygen administration with the subsequent development of RLF. There is no doubt that oxygen, either alone or in combination with as yet unidentified specific tissue factors (as seems more likely), is an etiologic agent in the production of RLF. On the other hand, only new blood vessels developing from undifferentiated mesoderm are susceptible to the administration of oxygen and to subsequent RLF development. If one accepts the fact that immature retinal vessels seem to be necessary for the development of RLF, then one must accept the fact that it is prematurity with immature vasculature that is responsible for RLF, not oxygen administration. The implications of this philosophy are obvious, but should not be interpreted as minimizing the role of oxygen in the pathologic process.

It has been shown adequately that fetal age, birth weight, and crown-to-heel length are inadequate predictors of gestational age. That is, diabetic mothers may have babies of high birth weight but with a relatively low gestational age; or smoking mothers may have infants with a low birth weight or a small crown-to-heel length but who are of a normal gestational age. Several criteria have been incorporated to ascertain gestational age, which is a more reliable predictor of retinal vasculature maturity.

Retinal vascularization begins at the optic disc at 4 months of gestational age and is complete shortly before or shortly after birth in a full-term infant. The degree of vascularization varies with gestational age, of course, but also varies between eyes of the same patient. The initial process in retinal vascularization appears to be a budding-off of the hyaloid artery of the major retinal arterioles, but in fact, this budding develops from a sheet of undifferentiated mesenchymal cells that are programmed for vascular development. The advancing edge of these cells has been determined by Ashton to be relatively undifferentiated cells; whereas the trailing edge (the so-called rear guard) involves more differentiation, developing, and reorganizing into capillaries and subsequently into arterioles and venules. The developing vascular channels generally assume a pentagonal configuration. Pericytes are acquired by the vessels later in their development. Pericytes are relatively immune to oxygen administration, whereas the newly developed and developing endothelial cells are quite susceptible to oxygen administration.

Recognizing the importance of vascular maturity as far as susceptibility to RLF is concerned, Roth[38] looked at a number of babies in the high-risk and premature nurseries specifically to assess the degree of vascular development. Six hundred fifty-four eyes of 327 babies were examined, and the gestational age was determined at birth for these infants. In this sample, Roth found that the extent of retinal vascularization coincided with the relative maturity of the infant as determined by gestational age, and further, that infants over 38 weeks of age, as determined by these criteria, uniformly had mature retinal vasculature. He further determined that the infants with birth weights of 3 kg or more had mature vasculature. When he looked at the birth weights of infants without grouping these infants, however, he found that some infants had a mature vasculature at a low birth weight, whereas others had an immature retinal vasculature at a birth weight approaching that of 3 kg.

As mentioned above, vascular development proceeds from undifferentiated mesenchymal cells that are programmed for capillary development. Pressure, flow rate, and tissue factors induce subsequent restructuring into arteries and veins. In the pathologic process of RLF, however, oxygen and local tissue factors cause the mesenchymal cells to die or lose their orientation and the most recently developed capillaries to become obliterated. Pressure differentials (presumably) in the area of ongoing vascular development then lead to the formation of a mesenchymal arteriovenous shunt. Enough endothelial cells and undifferentiated mesenchymal cells may remain to form new capillary buds and new arterioles and veins, thus obliterating the shunt, leaving varying degrees of evidence of its prior existence. On the other hand, the shunt may persist for a time, with attempted new vessel formation from cells capable of this enterprise, which exist posterior to the shunt. Abnormal vessels may grow from the retina up into the vitreous with subsequent fracture, bleeding, fibrous ingrowth, and cicatricial contracture.

It seems reasonable to postulate that the advancing area of vascular development is in response to as yet undetermined, local tissue factors produced by, or associated with, relative hypoxia of that tissue. When oxygen is administered in excess of the local demand, either the cells that respond to a hypoxic state in the above described manner lose their orientation, their potential for future development is lost or retarded, or they die. Subsequent inadequate oxygen in the peripheral retinal tissues becomes a powerful stimulant for renewed vessel ingrowth, which must then be attempted with an inadequate substrate, which, in turn, leads to abnormal vessel development (although sometimes adequate to complete the vascularization process) or to greater degrees of abnormality, including those of neovascular tissue growing up into the vitreous. These new vessels are never normal, and intervessel capillaries are always deficient, even when the retina appears to have recovered from the initial disturbance.

190

Flynn[27] has described the differences between the normal vascularization of an immature retina and the vascularization occurring in a retina with developing RLF, and this description is restated as follows.

In the normal retina a fine line exists in the periphery, which separates the vascular from the avascular retina. No blood vessels can be seen to exist clinically or with the microscope in histology sections anterior to this line. There is a blend of vascular and avascular tissue without other distinctive area changes. Small arteries and veins lead to the area of active vascular development. On the other hand, in RLF cases, a coarse, thickened line is present at the area of vascular activity. Abrupt changes seem to occur in this area, and large feeder vessels can be demonstrated leading to this area of activity. With fluorescein angiography, areas can be seen that represent shunts, the mesenchymal arteriovenous shunt being the first recognizable and pathognomonic sign of the presence of active RLF. When neovascularization takes place, it occurs posterior to the shunt. This neovascular tissue always leaks fluorescein. It appears that relatively differentiated cells in this area respond to peripheral tissue demands for oxygen in a more pathologic way than the cells in the immediate vicinity of the shunt where the substrate might have been more severely affected by the previous oxygen administration. This new vascular tissue is, as stated above, always abnormal. Regression of the pathologic process occurs in an estimated 85% of cases, with 15% going on to cicatrization. When regression occurs, abnormal vessel development can be demonstrated by fluorescein angiography. The abnormal vessels are those vessels extending beyond the area of the previously recognized shunt. These vessels are seen to have no polygonal network, with few capillaries existing between feeder vessels. Vessels often end in abrupt terminations, either club-shaped or frondlike, and may appear unusually straight or with clearly abnormal branching.

When cicatrization ensues, the only sign of the previous pathologic process may be small areas of chorioretinal pigment disturbance in the temporal periphery of the fundus. These areas may be associated with small localized areas of retinal detachment, and, although vessels in the vicinity are abnormal if examined using fluorescein angiography, obvious, clinical evidence of vessel abnormality may not be apparent. In our experience, most significant degrees of RLF are associated with the presence of significant myopia in the affected eye. Grades I and II RLF may be compatible with good vision (20/40 or better), whereas grade III usually has a visual acuity of 20/50 or less. Grade IV is associated with further reductions in vision, and grade V is usually associated with no better than light perception.

The great variability of this disorder, not only in terms of infants of different gestational ages and varying degrees of oxygen administration, but also between the eyes of the same individual, has made the management of these cases extremely difficult. In our series of cases, we have one set of twins with three of the four eyes having grade IV or V RLF, but the fourth eye is essentially normal. Other authors have reported similar experiences. Recognizing this individual susceptibility has made the prevention of RLF by monitoring oxygen administration frustrating and, to date, a procedure of less than 100% effectiveness. No one questions the toxicity of oxygen to susceptible tissues.

Certain experimental work, along with the extrapolation of clinical data, suggests that an oxygen level of 160 mm Hg or more is definitely toxic to immature vasculature within a 6-hour period. The susceptible cells seem to resist this toxicity for a time, but 6 hours or more at this level can initiate the process. Intermittent reductions in oxygen exposure are expected to be beneficial. Constant monitoring of oxygen saturation lowers the incidence of RLF but does not prevent it entirely. Many cases have now been reported in which RLF (or changes indistinguishable from those of RLF) occurred in retinas of mature infants, in infants who did not receive supplemental oxygen, and indeed, in infants in whom the presence of cardiovascular malformations precluded even normal oxygen levels in the eye. Other cases are reported where susceptible infants had as many as 200 samples of Pa_{O_2} measured every 1 to 3 hours with the appropriate regulation of oxygen concentration, but who developed cicatricial RLF despite this vigorous attention to oxygen levels. Skin electrodes with constant oxygen monitoring may enhance the prevention of this condition, but it remains to be seen whether RLF is an entirely preventable disorder. Although the prevention of excessive oxygen availability seems to be the only available clinical tool at this time, this alone is not adequate for the prevention of all cases of RLF. Local tissue availability of oxygen and the as yet unidentified but surely present tissue factors that play a role in vascular development are equally important.

Infants with exchange transfusions because of incompatibility have been suspected to be more susceptible to RLF, perhaps because the adult hemoglobin makes oxygen more available to those peripheral tissues in which susceptibility is so important.

Anesthetic administration to premature infants also should be undertaken with caution because of the probabilities of achieving high Pa_{O_2} levels during the administration of supplemental oxygen.

Finally, additional information provided by Roth[38] suggests that the incidence of pupillary membranes and hyaloid remnants is roughly correlated with the presence of immature retinal vasculature. The presence of these membranes might alert the pediatrician or family practitioner to the potential for RLF in those cases. The high-risk infant is certainly that infant suffering repeated episodes of respiratory distress who weighs 1,600 gm or less.

Treatment

Attempts have been made to treat active RLF with cryotherapy applied over the hypoxic retinal area. Success has been reported in a few cases, but in other similar cases the fellow eye has been observed to proceed to healthy development *without* treatment. Since some RLF eyes may be harmed by cryotherapy, the ultimate role of this treatment is unknown. Retinal detachment can occur in older patients with RLF and can be treated successfully with standard techniques.

PLATE 8-4

A Extent of retinal vascularization according to gestational age in months.
B Active retrolental fibroplasia.
Class:

(O) Incompletely vascularized retina, constricted arterioles.
(I) Incompletely vascularized retina, dilated veins.
(II) Peripheral hemorrhages, localized detachment.
(III) More extensive retinal detachment.
(IV) Nearly complete retinal detachment.
(V) Total retinal detachment.

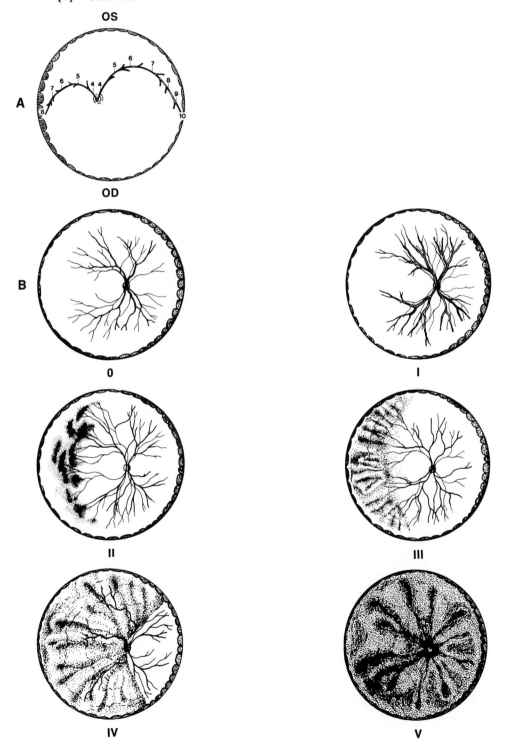

PLATE 8-4

PLATE 8-5

Cicatricial retrolental fibroplasia (retinopathy of prematurity).
A *Stage:*
  (I) Chorioretinal scarring in the periphery.
  (II) Chorioretinal scarring in the periphery, some with surrounding retinal detachment.
  (III) Traction on the temporal retina with a fold through the macula.
  (IV) Temporal retinal detachment.
  (V) Total retinal detachment.
B Patient demonstrates clinical appearance of grade V ROP.
C After bilateral enucleation for severe ocular pain.
D Stage II ROP in the right eye, vision 20/30.
E Stage III ROP in the left eye, vision 20/200.
F Periphery of the left eye demonstrating traction fold.

RETINOBLASTOMA

Retinoblastoma is the most common intraocular neoplasm in childhood, occurring approximately once in 25,000 live births. Retinoblastoma may arise as a somatic mutation, in which case the disease is unilateral and is not transmitted, or it may arise as a genetic mutation, in which case it is nearly always bilateral and is transmitted as an autosomal dominant disorder with about 80% penetrance. Retinoblastoma is highly malignant and only rarely do untreated cases survive. The tumor arises from cells of the retina of photoreceptor origin. Some retinoblastoma cells develop as rings around a central lumen, thus forming rosettes or fleurettes, depending on their degree of differentiation. Because of rapid intraocular growth, these tumors are frequently necrotic and therefore have a tendency to accumulate calcium. The tumor may spread by direct extension if the scleral shell is penetrated, or it may spread to the central nervous system, bone marrow, or viscera by blood-borne metastases.

Diagnosis

Retinoblastoma is usually diagnosed by its typical clinical appearance. The tumors are buff-colored with overlying vessels, and they usually occur in children between 6 months and 2 years of age. In our experience, bilateral tumors are diagnosed earlier, with the average age being about 1 year; and unilateral tumors are diagnosed later, with the average age being about 2½ years.

Retinoblastoma may occur as a single tumor in one eye, or as multiple tumors in both eyes. Unilateral retinoblastoma often presents as a single, large tumor, occupying one quarter to one half the vitreous space. Unilateral retinoblastoma usually arises from a single somatic mutation, but it may be hereditary. Bilateral retinoblastoma may occur in a variety of configurations, from a large tumor in one eye and a single small tumor in the second eye, to large tumors filling both eyes. Between these two extremes of presentation is the most common presentation of bilateral retinoblastoma, that is, a large tumor in one eye with multiple smaller tumors averaging 1 to 3 disc diameters in the second eye. About 40% of all patients with retinoblastoma have bilater-

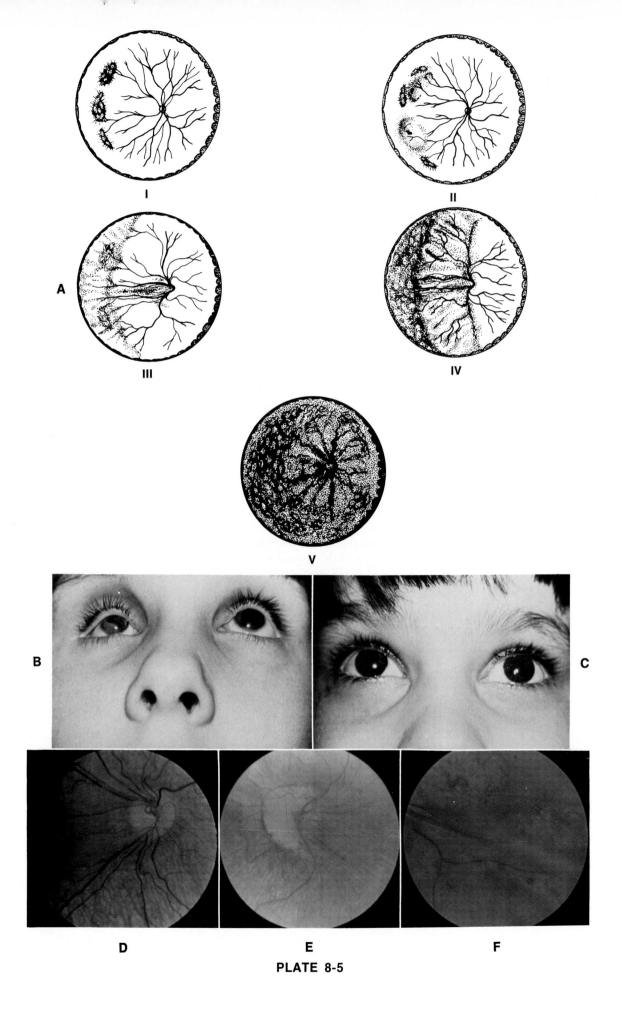

PLATE 8-5

al involvement. The single most important requisite for the diagnosis of retinoblastoma is an examination by an experienced examiner. No other diagnostic test is more valid than this observation. The findings of intraocular calcium on a bone-free x-ray film and increased aqueous/serum ratios of lactic dehydrogenase have been suggested as useful diagnostic tools but remain unreliable tests. Ultrasound examination with the A-scan or B-scan can be helpful, and stereoscopic photographs are useful, but these examinations are all adjunctive and cannot replace visual examination by an experienced observer.

Diagnostic workup

The diagnostic work-up of a patient suspected of having retinoblastoma should be individualized. In a case of unilateral retinoblastoma, in which useful vision is precluded in the involved eye, the patient should have an enucleation of this eye as soon as possible. The diagnosis must be confirmed by histologic examination. If the tumor appears on histologic section to be confined to the eye, a chest film, complete blood count, and urinalysis may be an adequate workup. On the other hand, in cases in which there is more concern about the possibility of metastasis, a more extensive workup should be done, which includes a metastatic bone survey, bone scan, bone marrow examination, and lumbar puncture with histologic study of the spinal fluid. These examinations are best carried out with the cooperation of a pediatric hematologist-oncologist. Unfortunately, if metastic retinoblastoma is found, even heroic methods of treatment have been generally unsuccessful in sustaining life for more than 1 year.

If any evidence of abnormal development suggestive of a chromosomal abnormality is present, the patient is referred for a genetic workup in order to evaluate the possibility of the presence of a 13q deletion syndrome or other chromosomal abnormalities. Research in these areas may lead eventually to chromosomal identification of many genetic carriers of retinoblastoma.

Treatment

Retinoblastoma is treated by enucleation of the visually compromised eye and by external irradiation to any tumors that remain in the fellow eye. On the average, 4,000 rads are delivered by the linear accelerator in doses of 200 rads per day for 20 sessions. Patients are anesthetized or sedated as required for these treatments under the supervision of the radiation oncologist. During the course of radiation and afterward, the eyes are examined, and any new tumor growth is treated on an individual basis. Anteriorly located retinal tumors are treated with cryotherapy. In some cases, tumors at or behind the equator can be reached with the cryoprobe only after an incision is made in the conjunctiva. Each tumor so treated is completely engulfed in an ice ball two or three times. Lesions that are too far posterior for cryotherapy, even with conjunctival incision, are treated by placing a ring of xenon arc photocoagulation around the tumor and then by treating the surface of the tumor. Cryotherapy is more effective than photocoagulation because the lightly colored tumors reflect rather than absorb heat from the photocoagulation. The theoretical objection to photocoagulation (that is, destruction of Bruch's membrane with removal of this barrier to tumor extension) has not been a recognized clinical entity in our series of patients so treated.

Tumors that are resistant to external beam radiation or that project too high above the retina to be engulfed by cryotherapy are treated with placement of a cobalt-60 plaque. The dose of radiation to be delivered by this plaque must be individualized and is calculated by the radiation physicist based on estimates of tumor size. The plaque is placed adjacent to the tumor and is removed several days later when the appropriate dose of radiation has been delivered.

Follow-up

The follow-up of a retinoblastoma patient requires diligence and teamwork. Patients with unilateral disease are seen at 1-month intervals for 3 to 4 months, at 2- to 3-month intervals for 6 months, then at 6-month intervals until they are 5 years old, and at yearly intervals after that. In our series, unilateral retinoblastoma, except in genetic cases seen very early in life, never become bilateral. Other authors have reported a delayed appearance of retinoblastoma in the fellow eye. Patients with bilateral retinoblastoma are seen at 1-month intervals for 6 months; then, if the condition is stable, at 2- or 3-month intervals for the next year, at 6-month intervals until age 5, and at 1-year intervals after that. Of course, the follow-up of bilateral retinoblastoma must be highly individualized, because prompt, effective local treatment of recurrent or newly developed tumors is necessary to save both sight and life. We suggest that regional comprehensive retinoblastoma treatment centers should be established so that patients can be followed on a regular basis without imposing undue hardships and unnecessary delays in examination and treatment because of distance. It is likely that travel hardships might reduce the flexibility of follow-up and thereby increase the possibility of a tumor becoming out of control.

Heredity

Once the diagnosis of retinoblastoma has been made and treatment is well under way, it is the responsibility of the treating physician to perform a retinal examination of family members at risk and provide the patient's family with complete, accurate information regarding the heredity of the disorder.

Classification

Retinoblastoma is classified according to its clinical presentation, treatment requirements, and the possibilities of salvaging vision. As a general rule, an eye with a large tumor or multiple large tumors with the macula involved is enucleated promptly if the other eye has any potential for useful vision. The reason for this is that it seems to be unwarranted to attempt to save a severely handicapped eye that on the one hand provides little if any useful vision and on the other hand harbors a tumor that may prove lethal if metastases develop. A second eye or any eye in which the macula is not involved is treated vigorously in an attempt to salvage vision. As a guideline, it is more important to sustain life than it is to sustain vision at the eventual expense of life. The classification that follows is a departure from the Reese-Ellsworth Classification and is based on treatment requirements.

PLATE 8-6

A Class I. The most common presentation of *unilateral* retinoblastoma is a large (10 or more disc diameter) tumor involving the macula and projecting into the vitreous. These patients have strabismus, leukocoria, or both. These patients are treated with enucleation of the involved eye and careful examination and observation of the fellow eye. No special workup is undertaken, and no prophylactic treatment is directed toward the uninvolved eye. We have never seen a retinoblastoma lesion develop in the initially uninvolved eye of a patient who had *advanced* unilateral disease (not the neonate with hereditary retinoblastoma).

B Class Ia. A rare presentation of unilateral retinoblastoma is a small (2 to 6 disc diameter) lesion not involving the macula. We have seen this presentation in three of 50 patients. Two of these cases were hereditary, and the patients subsequently (within weeks) developed lesions in the other eye in spite of external beam irradiation. The other patient had treatment begun with external beam irradiation. However, after approximately 800 rads had been given, the patient developed a total retinal detachment, and the eye was enucleated.

C Class II. A common presentation of bilateral retinoblastoma is a large (10 disc diameter or larger) lesion involving the macula and projecting into the vitreous in one eye and a solitary small- to medium-sized (2 to 5 disc diameter) lesion in the periphery of the second eye. These patients are treated with enucleation of the more involved eye and external beam irradiation totalling 4,000 rads to the fellow eye.

D Class IIa. Bilateral retinoblastoma rarely presents with small (2 to 5 disc diameter) solitary or multiple tumors in the periphery or extramacular areas of each eye. We have seen this type of presentation in two patients with hereditary retinoblastoma, who were examined because of a high degree of suspicion. It is unlikely that such a diagnosis would be made in a sporadic case except fortuitously. When a case such as this is seen, external irradiation should be applied to both eyes.

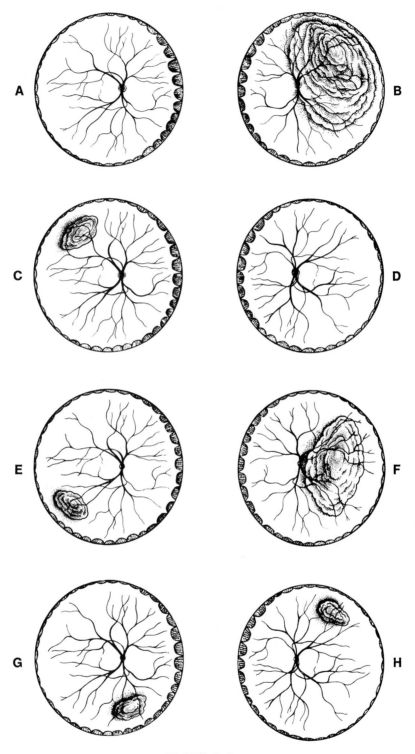

PLATE 8-6

PLATE 8-7

A Clinical appearance of class III retinoblastoma **(1)** in primary position and **(2)** in right gaze.

B Enucleated globe, class III retinoblastoma.

C Second eye of a Class II patient **(1)** before and **(2)** after treatment with 4,000 rads external beam irradiation and photocoagulation.

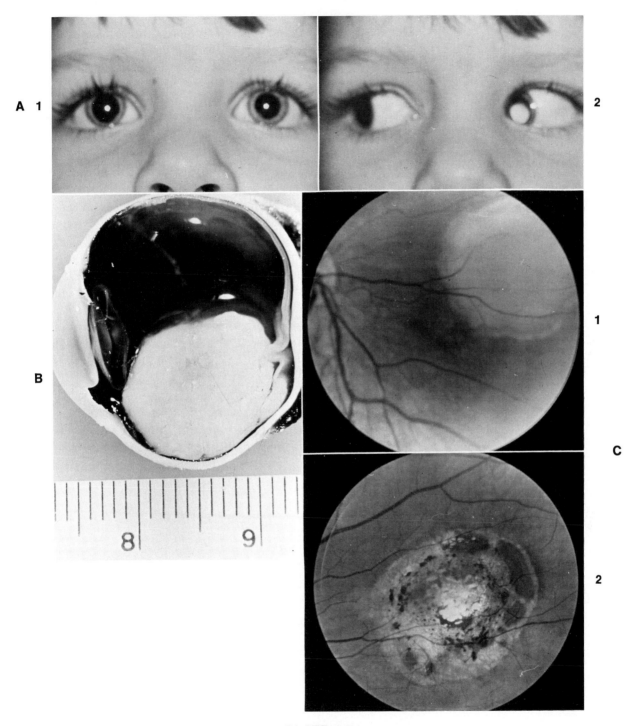

PLATE 8-7

PLATE 8-8

A Class III. The most common presentation of *bilateral* retinoblastoma occurs with one eye containing a large (10 disc diameter or more) tumor involving the macula and projecting into the vitreous, and the second eye having two or more small (2 to 5 disc diameter) tumors in the periphery or the posterior pole but not involving the macula or optic nerve. These patients are treated with enucleation of the more involved eye and 4,000 rads external beam irradiation to the remaining eye. During and after the course of irradiation, the treated eye is watched for the behavior of the treated tumors and for the development of any new tumors. If new tumors develop or if existing tumors enlarge during the course of irradiation, they are treated with cryotherapy, which consists of freezing until the entire tumor is engulfed in the ice ball. A two- or three-freeze technique is usually employed. After the irradiation is complete, careful follow-up is carried out, with frequent retinal examinations and local treatment with cryotherapy or photocoagulation as necessary.

B Class IV. In a more advanced type of bilateral retinoblastoma, one eye contains a large (10 disc diameter or more) tumor involving the macula and projecting into the vitreous and the second eye has a single or multiple tumors with at least one tumor in the posterior pole adjacent to or overriding the optic nerve head. The latter tumors may be difficult to treat, and on two occasions we have found it necessary to enucleate a second eye because such a tumor did not respond to irradiation and could not be controlled by local treatment.

C Class V. In bilateral retinoblastoma both retinas may be completely or nearly completely involved with tumor, and both vitreous cavities may be filled or nearly filled with tumor. We have treated three such cases with bilateral enucleation. In two cases the enucleations were done at the same operation, after we obtained frozen-section histologic confirmation that the tumor was retinoblastoma.

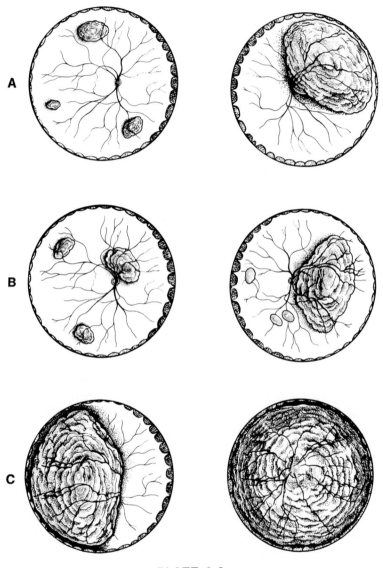

PLATE 8-8

PLATE 8-9

A Bilateral class V retinoblastoma **(1)** before and **(2)** after enucleation.
B Typical appearance of globes enucleated for class V retinoblastoma.

RETINAL DYSTROPHIES
Best vitelliform degeneration

Vitelliform retinal degeneration initially appears as a yellowish, smooth, dome-shaped, subretinal lesion of the macula. It is usually first noted as an incidental finding when the patient is between the ages of 5 and 15 years. Visual acuity is amazingly good in most cases, being 20/20 during this "sunny side up" phase. During the second to fourth decade, the yellow cyst may take on a scrambled appearance, and when this occurs, vision is reduced severely. The loss of vision can be sudden. Vitelliform retinal degeneration is transmitted as an autosomal dominant disorder. It is usually bilateral. The ERG is normal, but the EOG light rise/dark fall ratio is reduced, even in the carriers who have normal-appearing fundi. EOG testing should be carried out on all suspected carriers, and when an abnormality is found, they should be advised of the possibility of passing on the trait.

Fundus flavimaculatus

Fundus flavimaculatus is characterized by soft, yellow amorphous flecks randomly scattered throughout the fundus. The flecks change in appearance from one examination to another. This disorder has been further classified to include those cases of macular degeneration with peripheral lesions known as Stargardt disease. Thus, macular degeneration may or may not be a prominent part of this picture. This disorder usually is recessively inherited, but occasional dominant inheritance, occurs.

Symptoms usually appear in the first or second decade, usually depending upon whether or not the macula is involved early or late. Fluorescein angiography is helpful for early diagnosis. The ERG is generally normal, as is the EOG. Color vision is usually normal unless the macular disease is advanced. Night vision is usually normal.

Stargardt disease

Stargardt disease is a slowly progressive macular dystrophy beginning at about the time of puberty. The initial clinical appearance is that of a loss of luster of the normal macular reflex. This progresses slowly, with pigmentary mottling and occasionally with hemorrhages. Vision decreases slowly but steadily, and by the fourth decade acuity is 20/200. The peripheral retina is not destroyed, and total blindness does not occur. The pathologic process involves destruction of the retinal pigment epithelium and visual cells primarily in the area of the macula and posterior pole. The condition is transmitted as an autosomal recessive disorder, but occasionally autosomal dominant cases do occur. This disorder is now best classified as fundus flavimaculatus with macular involvement.

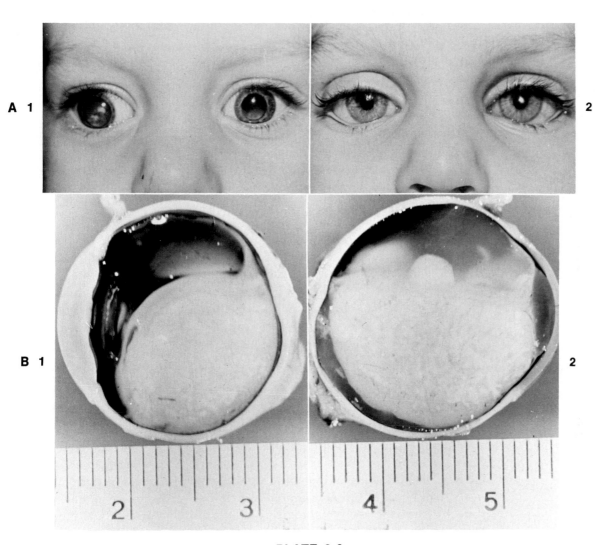

PLATE 8-9

Leber amaurosis

Children who have Leber amaurosis generally have symptoms attributable to absent vision from birth. Thus, they may have nystagmus and poor or absent following movements. The pupils may react poorly to light. The fundus may appear normal in early months but may become granular or stippled later. The optic nerves may be slightly pale. Later changes typical of retinitis pigmentosa may appear. The ERG response is extinguished. Inheritance is generally autosomal recessive.

Batten-Mayou disease

Batten-Mayou disease is one of the progressive neuronal ceroid-lipofuscinoses. The onset is insidious, but the course is progressively downhill, with mental and visual deterioration. Several types have been described.

The ocular findings include a peculiar metallic appearance of the macula, pale discs, thin pigment epithelium, and attenuation of the vasculature. Color vision may degenerate as the macula is affected.

Diagnosis may be assisted by the findings of a reduced ERG response, abnormal vacuolated peripheral leukocytes, or ceroid bodies in skeletal muscles (using electron microscopy).

Choroideremia

Choroideremia is a sex-linked recessive disorder characterized by a gradual degeneration of the outer retinal layer producing a creamy white appearance to affected areas. It generally begins in the periphery, progressing toward the disc. The retinal vessels retain a relatively normal appearance until late in the disease, as does the optic nerve head. The ERG b wave is diminished early, and may become extinguished late.

Gyrate atrophy

Gyrate atrophy is a slowly progressive choroidal disease in which loss of the choroid, pigment epithelium, and retina occurs. The process begins in the midperiphery and eventually involves the entire retina. The last area involved is the macula. Night blindness and field loss are early signs caused by loss of the retinal periphery, but severe visual loss occurs later in the disease. Optic atrophy, myopia, and cataracts may accompany the retinal signs. Abnormally high levels of serum ornithine have been found, and when this is confirmed by enzyme assay, the diagnosis is established. Heredity is probably autosomal recessive, since the family members have been known to possess intermediate high levels of ornithine and respond abnormally to loading doses of ornithine.

PLATE 8-10

A Best vitelliform macular dystrophy.
B Retinitis pigmentosa.
C Early choroideremia.
D Gyrate atrophy.

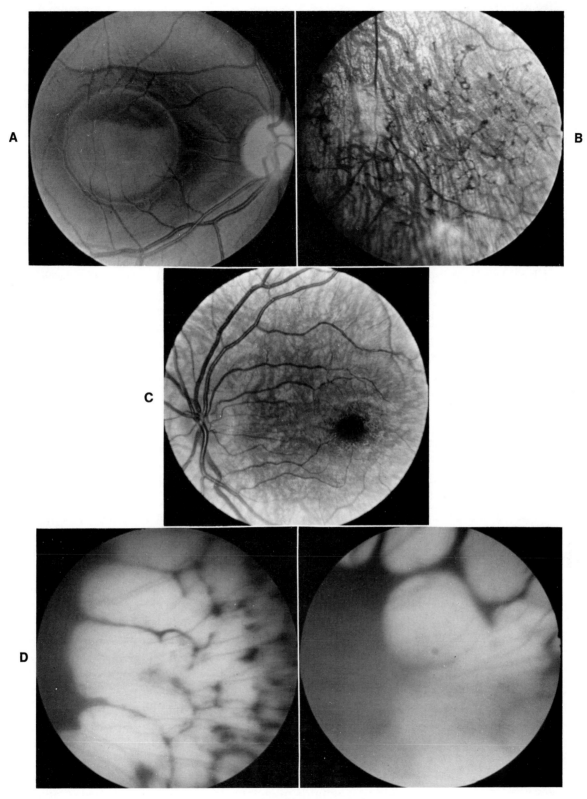

PLATE 8-10

207

Retinitis pigmentosa

A large group of related diseases that have systemic as well as ocular manifestations have in common a progressive deterioration of the retinal pigment epithelium and outer segments of the rods and cones, with subsequent loss of function of visual cells. As the disease progresses, varying amounts of pigment dispersion are seen in the retina. This accumulation usually takes on the configuration of bone spicules. This pigmentation is seen most often in the mid periphery of the retina. Other typical changes include a waxy pallor of the optic nerve and attenuation of the retinal vessels. The most important finding in this disease group (which from the ocular standpoint is classified as *retinitis pigmentosa*) is that of a reduced or extinguished ERG response. This finding is present even before visual symptoms develop or clinically visible retinal changes occur. When retinitis pigmentosa in any of its manifestations is suspected, a flat or extinguished ERG response confirms the diagnosis. Progressive deterioration in visual function can be expected. Volumes have been written dealing with differential diagnosis, classification, etiology, and heredity of the retinitis pigmentosis disorders; therefore, anything but a superficial review of these entities is beyond the scope of this book.

It is important to look for associated signs or symptoms in the patient with retinitis pigmentosa. That is, does the patient also have a hearing defect? Does he have neurologic or cardiovascular disease? Is there any evidence of dermatitis or gastrointestinal symptoms? If associated, significant abnormalities are present, it is probable that the disorders are related and that the retinitis pigmentosa is a part of a larger picture, which can be recognized and categorized.

Retinitis pigmentosa is an inherited, degenerative disorder with ominous visual implications. The onset may be early in life or in the second or third decade. Early symptoms may be unrecognized by the patient, who has no reason to suspect an ocular problem. Night blindness, loss of equatorial visual field, constriction of fields, and eventual blindness may result. Early signs of retinitis pigmentosa are the bone-corpuscle accumulations of pigment in the equatorial regions of the eye, attenuated retinal arterioles, pale, yellow discs, and posterior subcapsular cataract.

Inheritance is autosomal recessive, autosomal dominant, or sex-linked recessive.

The ERG response is markedly abnormal or extinguished.

Dark adaptation also is markedly abnormal. Patients with retinitis pigmentosa in which the diagnosis is readily established by means of the family history, physical findings, and abnormal ERG response are counseled as to the mode of probable inheritance of their disorder and as to the expected role of progression, taking the most optimistic course when possible. Sunglasses are offered for the theoretical retardation of photoreceptor breakdown by decreased light exposure, although it is emphasized that their effectiveness has not been proved.

More difficult classes of patients exist, however, who have retinitis pigmentosa–like conditions, retinitis pigmentosa syndromes, or who have "atypical retinitis pigmentosa." Most disorders causing widespread retinal pigment disturbances that superficially suggest retinitis pigmentosa have a normal or nearly normal ERG response, thus ruling out typical retinitis pigmentosa. Congenital rubella, viral retinopathy, and so on can be ruled out by their atypical appearance, combined with the presence of a normal ERG response.

Other syndromes associated with abnormal ERGs and a picture of retinitis pigmentosa include the following.

I. Disorders associated with degenerative central nervous system disease

    A. Ataxia syndromes

        1. Bassen-Kornzweig syndrome: abetalipoprotinemia, acanthocytosis; autosomal recessive

        2. Merzbacher-Pelizaeus disease: mental deterioration and spasticity; sex-linked recessive

        3. Flynn-Aird syndrome: cataracts, mental deterioration, seizures; autosomal dominant

        4. Friedreich ataxia: posterior column disease, nystagmus, optic atrophy; autosomal recessive

        5. Hallervorden-Spatz syndrome: basal ganglia symptoms, mental deterioration, and early death; autosomal recessive

        6. Hallgren syndrome: deafness, mental retardation, cataract, and nystagmus; autosomal recessive

        7. Hereditary olivopontocerebellar degeneration: athetosis, slurred speech; autosomal recessive

    B. Other central nervous system disorders with retinitis pigmentosa – like retinopathy

        1. Ceroid lipofuscinosis: mental deterioration and epilepsy; autosomal recessive

        2. Laurence-Moon-Biedl-Bardet syndrome: mental retardation, obesity, hypogenitalism, polydactyly; autosomal recessive

II. Disorders associated with deafness

    A. Usher syndrome: autosomal recessive

    B. Cockayne syndrome: dwarfism and mental retardation; autosomal recessive

    C. Hallgren syndrome (see above)

    D. Laurence-Biedl syndrome: autosomal recessive (see above)

    E. Ophthalmoplegia-plus syndrome

    F. Alström syndrome: obesity, diabetes mellitus, nystagmus; autosomal recessive

    G. Refsum disease: autosomal recessive (see below)

III. Mucopolysaccharidosis

    A. Type I_H, Hurler syndrome: autosomal recessive
       Type I_S Scheie syndrome: autosomal recessive

    B. Type II, Hunter syndrome: sex-linked recessive

    C. Type III, Sanfilippo syndrome: autosomal recessive

    D. Type IV, Morquio syndrome: autosomal recessive

IV. Disorders associated with dermatologic problems

    A. Flynn-Aird syndrome: skin changes (nonspecific)

B. Refsum disease: excoriation, polyneuritis, increased plasma phytanic acid; autosomal recessive
C. Rud syndrome: ichthyosis; heredity unknown
V. Disorders associated with renal problems
A. Saldmo syndrome: nephropathy, cerebellar ataxia, and skeletal abnormalities; autosomal recessive
B. Fanconi syndrome: renal failure; autosomal recessive
VI. Disorders associated with muscle, skeletal, structural, or cardiac disorders
A. Ophthalmoplegia plus: may have heart block
B. Muscular dystrophy: cataracts
C. Kartagener syndrome: dextrocardia, sinusitis, bronchiectasis
D. Turner syndrome: XO chromosome pattern, short stature, low hairline, webbed neck
E. Mucopolysaccharidoses (see above)
F. Laurence-Biedl syndrome (see above)
G. Cockayne syndrome (see above)
VII. Disorders secondary to infection (ERG normal or only mildly affected)
A. Syphilis
B. Viremia
C. Bacteremia
VIII. Disorders associated with drugs
A. Vitamin A toxicity
B. Chloroquine toxicity
C. Chlorpromazine toxicity
D. Thioridazine toxicity

A specific diagnosis facilitates understanding the patient's symptoms and allows the progression or lack of progression of retinitis pigmentosa to be anticipated. The physician can then counsel the patient as to educational goals, realistic work goals, and family planning. Secondary causes of retinitis pigmentosa–like syndrome may be treatable by withholding medication, dietary management, or specific antiviral or antibacterial therapy. As more of these disorders are found to have specific enzymatic or genetic defects, more specific therapy will become available.

Congenital stationary night blindness

Congenital stationary night blindness generally is inherited as a sex-linked recessive disorder, especially when associated with significant myopia, although all forms of inheritance have been described. Nystagmus may be present. The ERG may be diagnostic in that the dark- and light-adapted wave form have equal intensities.

PHAKOMATOSES
Sturge-Weber syndrome

The most obvious feature of Sturge-Weber syndrome is the facial cutaneous angiomatosis (flame nevus) that occurs unilaterally in the upper part of the face in the area innervated by the trigeminal nerve. Intracerebral angiomas may cause epilepsy, and trabecular involvement causes glaucoma. Choroidal angiomas impart a darkened appearance to the fundi. No treatment is successful for this condition, although topical and systemic medication to reduce aqueous production and cryotherapy are helpful.

Von Hippel-Lindau disease

Von Hippel-Lindau disease is characterized by a globular, reddish mass in the retina, which may be smaller than the disc, or it may occupy a 10 disc diameter area of the retina and project into the vitreous a like amount. The tumor is vascular with a large feeder artery and accompanying vein. This condition is transmitted as an autosomal dominant disorder with incomplete penetrance. It may be treated successfully in some cases with photocoagulation. Intracranial angiomatosis in this disease may require treatment in specific cases.

Neurofibromatosis (von Recklinghausen disease)

The most common fundus lesion of neurofibromatosis is the marked papilledema associated with a glioma involving the optic nerve. Neurofibromas may involve the uveal tract, and (rarely) nodular white or yellow lesions occur in the retina. Skin lesion, both depigmented and hyperpigmented, are cutaneous manifestations of neurofibromatosis. Lesions involving the lids and orbit, choroidal lesions, iris nodules, increased visibility of corneal nerves, glaucoma, and meningeal lesions are all a part of this process, which is transmitted as an autosomal dominant trait.

Tuberous sclerosis

The fundus picture of tuberous sclerosis is that of multiple (one to five) yellowish or white, rounded or dimpled masses on or around the optic nerve head or in the posterior pole, generally about one disc diameter in size. These tumors are hamartomas made up of a proliferation of pleomorphic cells thought to be elements of glial cells. This process also goes on in the central nervous system, and progressive mental and physical deterioration precedes death, which usually occurs by the end of the third decade. Lesions occur over the bridge of the nose in a butterfly configuration in the form of 2- to 4-mm yellowish nodules, called adenoma sebaceum. The heredity of this condition is difficult to establish, because involved individuals tend to die or be institutionalized before the reproductive years, but studies of pedigrees have led to the conclusion that tuberous sclerosis may be transmitted as an irregular dominant trait with low penetrance.

STORAGE DISEASES
Carbohydrate and lipid metabolism and storage diseases

A wide variety of related diseases occur as the direct result of abnormalities in lipid and carbohydrate metabolism and result in the storage of both lipids and mucopolysaccharides. These diseases are associated with severe systemic manifestations, including mental retardation, and often result in early death. Lipid storage in ganglion cells, which leads to a "cherry-red" spot in the macula, is a common feature of many of the lipid metabolism and storage diseases. As with retinitis pigmentosa–related diseases, the lipid metabolism and storage diseases have been studied by many experts, who have accurately described, in detail, significant differences in many of these diseases; therefore, a large number of separate but similar conditions exist. The defect that ultimately produces the metabolic deficiency is a specific enzyme defect in each case. The specific enzyme defect can be suspected from the clinical picture of the disease; that is, a cherry-red spot and early mental and physical retardation in a child with an Ashkenazic Jewish ancestry, who after normal early development undergoes physical and mental deterioration, suggests a diagnosis of Tay-Sachs disease (hexosaminidase-A deficiency). This disease and others can be confirmed by urine tests or blood tests or both for specific enzyme deficiencies. Also, this disease and a host of other diseases with ocular and systemic manifestations can be diagnosed prenatally. This, of course, raises the possibility that pregnancy may be terminated if there is indication that the fetus is affected.

When retinitis pigmentosa or a storage disease is suspected, specific reference sources should be consulted for details of enzymatic identification.

Mucopolysaccharidoses

The mucopolysaccharidoses are a related group of storage diseases characterized by lysosomal enzyme deficiency, the excretion of heparatin, dermatin, or keratin in the urine, and by corneal clouding in the majority of cases (all except mucopolysaccharidosis, types II, III, and IV.

Cardiac, skeletal, and central nervous system abnormalities characterize many of the disorders. Distinction between the disorders must be made, because the prognosis, the complications, cardiac problems, and intelligence range vary widely, being relatively normal in some and markedly abnormal in others. Specific diagnosis can be established by demonstrating the abnormal mucopolysaccharide in the urine, by measuring the enzyme deficiencies, and by identifying the specific cardiac, skeletal, or central nervous system abnormalities present in individual patients. The inheritance pattern is autosomal recessive in all cases except Hunter syndrome, which is sex-linked recessive. No specific therapy is available for any of the disorders.[12,25,26]

Mucolipidoses

The mucolipidoses are a goup of related storage disorders that are characterized by the storage of lipid and mucopolysaccharide material. In addition to significant systemic manifestations, ocular findings of corneal clouding (as in the mucopolysaccharide disorders) and cherry-red spots (as in the sphingolipidoses) occur. Specific enzyme defects probably exist in all cases and have been identified in many. All the disorders in which a hereditary pattern has been established are inherited in an autosomal recessive pattern.

The mucolipidoses that have significant ocular findings follow.

1. G_{m_1} gangliosidosis type 1: corneal clouding and macular cherry-red spots appear in this disorder
2. Mucolipidosis type I: corneal opacities and macular cherry-red spots

3. Mucolipidosis type II: corneal opacities and macular cherry-red spots
4. Mucolipidosis type III: corneal clouding
5. Lipogranulomatosis: macular cherry-red spots
6. Sea-blue histiocyte syndrome: macular cherry-red spots

Sphingolipidoses

The sphingolipidoses are characterized by the storage of a lipid material and by the ocular findings of cherry-red spots. Physical and mental deterioration are frequent components of these disorders. All are inherited in an autosomal recessive fashion except for Fabry disease, which is a sex-linked recessive disorder and has ocular findings other than cherry-red spots.

1. G_{m_2} gangliosidosis type 1 (Tay-Sachs disease):
   Ocular findings: Macular cherry-red spots.
2. G_{m_2} gangliosidosis type II (Sandhoff disease)
   Ocular findings: occasional macular cherry-red spots.
3. Neuronal ceroid-lipofuscinosis (Batten-Mayou disease)
   Ocular findings: Beaten metal appearance to macular area, optic atrophy.
4. Essential lipid histiocytosis (Niemann-Pick disease)
   Ocular findings: macular cherry-red spot.
5. Angiokeratoma corporis diffusum (Fabry disease)
   Ocular findings: Whorllike corneal dystrophy, posterior spokelike cataract, and prominent conjunctival blood vessels.
6. Globoid leukodystrophy (Krabbe disease)
   Ocular findings: Optic atrophy and nystagmus.
7. Infantile metachromatic leukodystrophy
   Ocular findings: Macular cherry-red spot.

RETINAL DETACHMENT

Retinal detachment occurs infrequently in childhood. The most common cause of retinal detachment in children is trauma followed by those causes secondary to retinopathy of prematurity and to myopic changes. In childhood, the underlying cause of the detachment is probably more significant than the detachment itself, because the inciting cause usually bodes ill for the health of the eye. Diagnostic and therapeutic measures in pediatric retinal detachment are carried out in a manner similar to those in adults.

INFLAMMATORY DISEASES
Toxocara canis

Toxocara canis usually appears in the retina as a white, smooth, elevated lesion in the macula, papillomacular bundle, posterior pole of the eye, or in the retinal periphery. Vision, of course, is reduced when the lesion is located posteriorly, and strabismus is likely to occur secondary to the reduction in central vision. Children are affected beginning in the toddler years, and occasional instances of initial involvement in children up to age 10 years or older have occurred. A history of association with a puppy is common, but because of the ubiquitous occurrence of pets in our society, a pet in the patient's home is not always reported. The presence of the eggs of *Toxocara canis* in the soil may be of long duration. These lesions eventually regress to a "hard" fibrous appearance with a larger surrounding chorioretinal scar. Tracks of the mobile worm may be seen in the retina and vitreous; occasionally lesions may be located peripherally. A laboratory test, the *Enzyme Linked Immunosorbent Assay* (ELISA) test, is available. Eosinophilia of 3% to 12% may be seen in the peripheral blood with the initial parasitemia, but this is seldom present at the time of diagnosis of the ocular lesion. Usually eosinophilia is present only with the other human form of the disease that is caused by *Toxocara canis*, visceral larva migrans. Clinical diagnosis on the basis of the appearance of the lesion remains the best diagnosis technique. There is no specific treatment for retinal *Toxocara canis*, although systemic steroids may help in the acute inflammatory stage.

Toxoplasmosis

Toxoplasmic retinitis, caused by the *Toxoplasma gondii* protozoa, is acquired in utero through the placental circulation from an acutely affected mother. The principal retinal lesion is white, punched out, or depressed, and surrounded by heavy pigmentation. When active, inflammatory cells and haze are present in the vitreous; satellite lesions are also frequently seen. Heavy exudation may occur in the vitreous. Systemically these children may have cerebral calcification, convulsions, jaundice, and hepatosplenomegaly. Typically the retinal lesions are bilateral in children but unilateral in adults. Treatment is indicated in active disease, particularly if the macula is threatened. Treatment may consist of sulfa, pyrimethamine, and folinic acid, or clindamycin. Steroids alone may contribute to the activation of the disease.

Cytomegalic inclusion disease

The uveal tract is one of many organs affected by the cytomegalovirus, which passes transplacentally from apparently well mothers. Many affected fetuses are stillborn. The living child shows multiple areas of chorioretinitis, which may coalesce as the child grows older. Diagnosis is made by demonstrating cerebral calcification on x-ray film and by identifying cytomegalovirus from the urine, tears, conjunctival scraping, or cerebrospinal fluid. In some cases the disease may be modified by systemic steroids.

Metastatic retinitis

On rare occasions, infectious emboli may spread to the retina, causing a severe chorioretinitis and vitreous reaction. This usually follows an exanthematous or other systemic disease. The condition is bilateral but asymmetrical and occurs without local ocular precursors. It may be overlooked because of the significance of the systemic problem. The classical descriptions of meningococcemia adequately outline this event, but recently an increasing number of emboli to the eye in the presence of *Hemophilus influenzae* infection has been noted.

Peripheral uveitis

Peripheral uveitis is said to be the second most common type of juvenile uveitis. It begins in the 6- to 10-year-old child, with an insidious onset. It may be noticed as an incidental finding at routine examination, or the patient may complain of blurred vision. The most obvious clinical finding is the presence of a large number of cells in the anterior vitreous, which may be hazy. Examination of the peripheral retina with scleral depression reveals a whitish cottonlike "snowbank" over the ora seratta, usually inferiorly. The disease may smolder for many years and then subside. Steroids may or may not be helpful in the treatment of individual cases. In rare cases, a cyclitic membrane may develop. Another term for this condition is pars planitis.

PLATE 8-11

A Acute *Toxocara canis.*
B *Toxocara canis* with track.
C *Toxocara canis* with stalk.
D Snowbank lesion, peripheral uveitis.

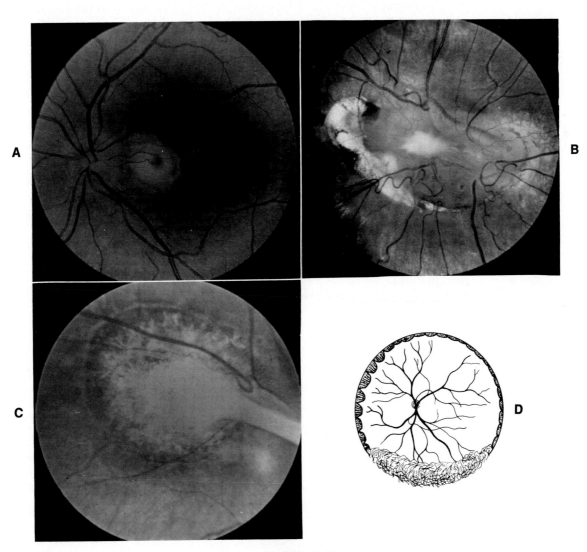

PLATE 8-11

OTHER PIGMENT ABNORMALITIES
Ocular albinism

Ocular albinism is inherited as a sex-linked and, rarely, autosomal recessive disorder and occurs, therefore, in males. Other signs of albinism are not present. The most important diagnostic test for this disorder is the examination of the mother's eyes, where one can see the mosaic pattern of pigmentation attributed to the dual genetic origin of the pigmented cell layer.

Children with ocular albinism have congenital nystagmus, blond fundi, and often a fair complexion early in life that darkens somewhat with age. These nonspecific findings make the diagnosis difficult in the absence of a family history or in the absence of the mother for examination. Skin biopsy demonstrating the presence of macromelanosomes can be helpful. The ERG amplitudes may be greater than normal.

These children are generally photophobic, and acuity is reduced. Nystagmus is present. Visual acuity is generally better than with universal albinism, often as good as 20/50.

Universal albinism

Deficient pigmentation involves not only the eye but the rest of the body and hair as well. If pigmentation is reduced but present, the condition is referred to as incomplete universal albinism. This disorder may also be divided as to the ability of tyrosinase-incubated hair bulbs to form melanin, thus producing tyrosinase-positive (melanin-forming) and tyrosinase-negative (non-melanin-forming) albinism. In general, tyrosinase-positive albinos have better acuity and tend to develop some pigmentation later in life. Individuals with tyrosinase-negative albinism have pendular nystagmus with visual acuity of 20/200 or worse. The maculas are generally poorly developed with no visible foveal reflex. Inheritance is generally autosomal recessive.

PLATE 8-12

A Pale irides.
B Hypopigmented fundi.

Choroidal nevus

Choroidal nevi are flat, grey to blue-grey, and have discrete borders. The lesions are stationary and usually are found posterior to the equator. These lesions produce no symptoms and do not ordinarily present a diagnostic problem in children.

Congenital melanosis of the retina (grouped pigmentation)

Congenital melanosis is a (usually) bilateral condition that is characterized by clusters of dark pigmentation, generally occurring in the peripheral retina, often in a sector. The shape of the pigment groups has been compared to a bear track. No visual impairment is produced, and no special significance is attached to this condition.

216

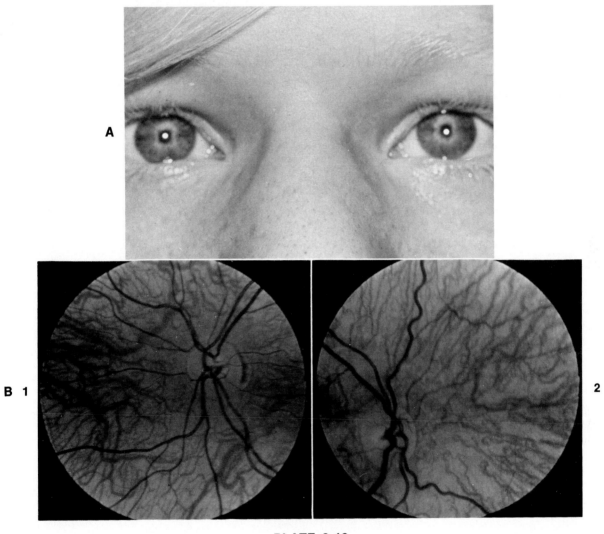

PLATE 8-12

217

Coats disease

Coats disease is characterized by exudation between the choroid and retina associated with telangiectasis of the retinal vessels. It is usually unilateral, occurring in males. The exudation may be mild and localized or may involve most of the retina, causing the vitreous cavity to be partially filled with a yellowish mass that may be confused with retinoblastoma. The disease may be relatively stable, or it may progress to severe visual impairment. Patients suspected of having Coats disease should be evaluated with fluorescein angiography and observed at regular intervals for evidence of progression. Treatment is not universally agreed upon, because some cases are not progressive. When treatment is carried out, it consists of photocoagulation of the telangiectatic areas.

Wyburn-Mason syndrome

Wyburn-Mason syndrome is characterized by a racemose angioma involving the vessels of the retina. Retinal involvement is extensive in some cases with the strikingly dilated and tortuous vessel and (when this is so) reduced vision. Telangiectatic vascular nevi affect the conjunctiva and skin around the eye, midbrain arteriovenous aneurysms are also present, and the orbit and optic nerve may also be involved. The condition is unilateral, and its inheritance is uncertain.

Chapter 9

THE ORBIT

The orbit is a conical bony recess of the skull with the base of the cone facing forward. The volume of the adult orbit is approximately 30 cc, and in the infant it is about one-half this size. Between birth and adulthood, the orbital volume increases proportionately with the growth of the face. The orbital contents comprise a variety of tissues, including fat, connective tissue, muscle, peripheral nerves and ganglia, blood vessels, glandular tissue, and, of course, a highly specialized complex neurosensory structure that is a direct extension of the brain—*the eye*. The orbital contents are subject to a wide variety of congenital and acquired diseases. Especially in the pediatric age group, orbital diseases, may be life threatening (orbital cellulitis, rhabdomyosarcoma) and demand prompt, accurate diagnosis and timely and appropriate treatment. Newer diagnostic techniques abound in ophthalmology, and the application of these techniques to the diagnosis of orbital disease certainly provides valuable help, but nowhere in ophthalmology are the old standby techniques of observation and palpation better applied.

The orbit is bordered by the ethmoid air cells medially. These are airified at birth and are separated from the orbit by a thin wall, the lamina papyracea. Sinus infection may spread through this wall, causing orbital cellulitis. The frontal sinus does not develop until about the second decade. The maxillary sinus is small but present at birth. Blowout fracture of the floor of the orbit does occur in childhood. The roof and lateral wall of the orbit are relatively thick and less frequently involved in trauma but may harbor metastatic disease or be the site of a histiocytosis X lesion.

The orbit is unique in that the rigid walls are noncompressible and, therefore, any new, space-occupying activity inside the confines of the orbit causes a forward displacement of the eye and orbital contents (proptosis). The manner in which the orbital contents come forward often can give a clue to the pathologic process within. If the eye comes straight forward and the mass is discrete, it may be in the muscle cone and may represent a hemangioma or a glioma of the optic nerve. If the eye is pushed out from the orbit and is dis-

219

placed laterally, medially, up or down, it is likely that the major orbital mass is outside the muscle cone and that it is located on the side opposite the direction of displacement. This occurs in rhabdomyosarcoma or subperiosteal metastatic neuroblastoma. The presence and degree of proptosis are determined by simple observation in the infant and child and are particularly evident if the child is viewed by the examiner looking down on the face while comparing the relative prominence of the two eyes.

Palpation, including attempts at retroplacement of the orbital contents, provides useful information about the size, shape, and consistency of the anteriorly placed orbital mass and about the compressibility of posteriorly placed masses. Of course, all necessary diagnostic tests should be carried out when indicated in the evaluation of orbital disease in childhood, but in an era of new, complicated, expensive diagnostic activity, it seems appropriate to stress the value and importance of physical examination carried out by observation and palpation. These observations may only precede other more involved tests, but they must never be ignored.

ORBITAL LESIONS
Relationship of location of orbital lesion and displacement of orbital contents

The eye and other orbital contents are usually displaced according to the location of the lesion. These findings can have significant diagnostic as well as therapeutic implications. Certain tumors are more likely to appear in particular parts of the orbit, and the surgical approach in the event that biopsy or excision is done will be influenced by the tumor location.

PLATE 9-1

A Configuration of the normal orbit.

B Proptosis that is straight forward and that causes the eye to bulge in the center of a symmetrically widened palpebral fissure usually is caused by a mass within the muscle cone or by an increase in volume of orbital contents as in pseudotumor or thyroid disease. The four rectus muscles joined by their intermuscular membrane provide a compartment that tends to limit migration of the expanding lesion.

C A mass lesion outside the muscle cone pushes the eye in the opposite direction and causes it to project forward.

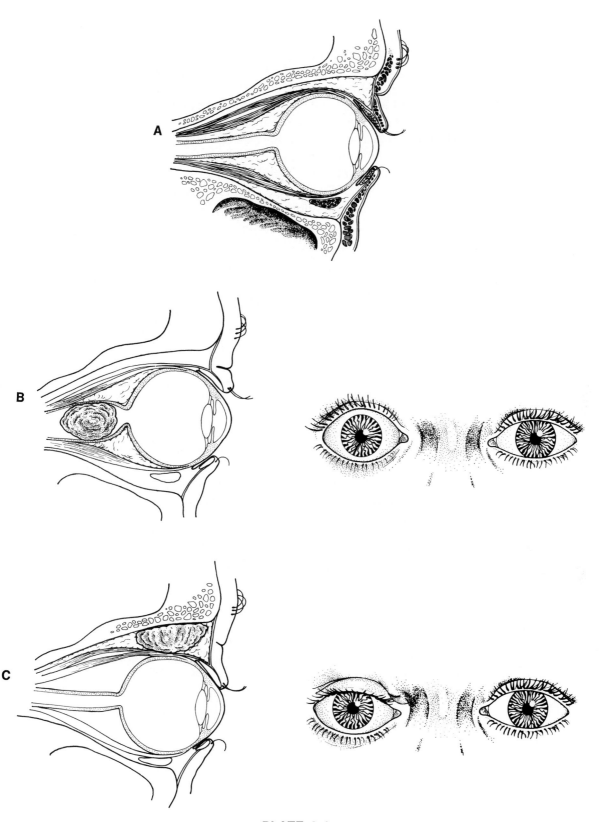

PLATE 9-1

PLATE 9-2

A A defect in the orbital wall that allows the escape of orbital contents, as with large blowout fractures of the orbital floor, causes diminished prominence of the globe and enophthalmos. The defect is accompanied by a narrowing of the palpebral fissure and often by limited ocular motility.

B An apparent proptosis can be produced by preseptal edema. The lids actually bulge forward, however, and the orbital contents are usually undisturbed. The orbital septum presents a formidable barrier to the spread of infection from without or within the orbit.

C Congenital shallow orbits produce proptosis because of a reduction in the bony orbital volume. The optic nerve may be placed on a stretch or compromised in the optic canal, producing optic atrophy.

Diagnostic techniques

Observation of the patient, particularly when done from above, provides ready comparison between the prominence of the two eyes and provides the basis for qualitative diagnosis of unilateral or in more obvious cases, bilateral proptosis. The examination can be further enhanced by the use of an exophthalmometer. This device sometimes cannot be accurately used on the infant or child. In that event, comparison of the palpebral fissures can provide an estimate of the relative amount of proptosis, particularly in unilateral cases.

The most common cause of unilateral proptosis reported in most series dealing with children is usually listed as dermoid cyst. In our experience these lesions are almost always anteriorly located outside the orbit, attached to the rim either superiorly and medially or superiorly and laterally. The lesions are fixed, firm, nearly round, and seem to be just under the skin, which indeed they are, although their deeper attachments may be extensive. B-scan ultrasonography can outline the shape and detail some of the characteristics of the orbital contents. A-scan ultrasonography provides information as to the size of the orbital mass and produces an indication of tissue type.

Films of the skull, including tomograms with special views of the optic canal, are useful to demonstrate bony orbital size, defects in the bony orbit, and symmetry between the two orbits and between the optic canals. Computerized axial tomography (CAT) is also an extremely useful tool in the study of orbital disease. The shape and location of orbital lesions can be determined with great accuracy, but care must be exercised in obtaining appropriate views both with and without contrast material for enhanced visibility.

Orbital venography employs x-ray studies of the orbit after the injection of radiopaque material into the frontal vein. Changes in the configuration and course of the superior ophthalmic vein provide indirect evidence of the presence of mass lesions in the orbit.

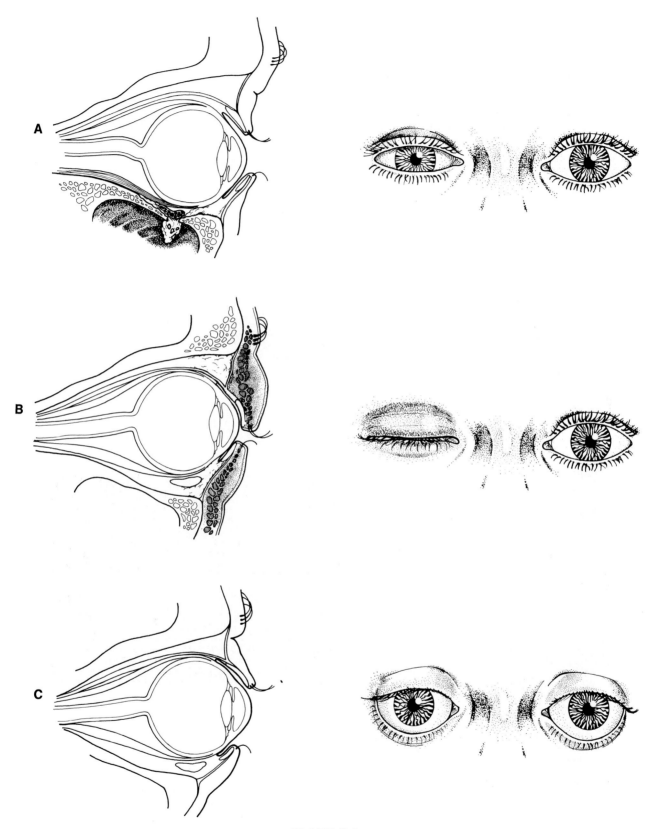

PLATE 9-2

PLATE 9-3

A **(1)** Unilateral proptosis of right eye viewed from above. **(2)** Bilateral un-
equal proptosis viewed from above.
B A large dermoid cyst of the lateral orbital rim.
C B-scan ultrasonography provides a two-dimensional view of the orbital
contents.
D A-scan ultrasonography provides a picture of tissue reflectivity in the orbit.
E CAT scan of a patient with proptosis of the right eye.
F Bone scan shows increased metabolic activity in the anterior orbit.

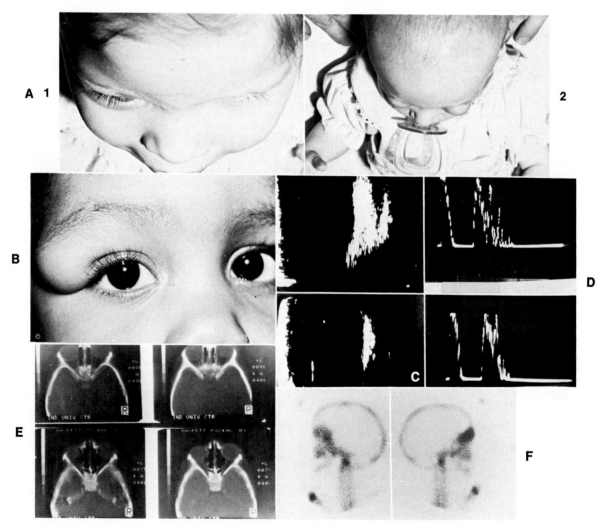

PLATE 9-3

Classification of orbital disease in childhood

The etiologies of disorders involving the orbit may be classified as follows:

Developmental
  Dermoid cysts
  Craniofacial syndromes
  Microphthalmos with cyst
  Teratomas
  Encephalocele
  Infantile cortical hyperostosis
Neoplastic
  Rhabdomyosarcoma
  Metastatic neuroblastoma
  Retinoblastoma
  Lymphoma
  Leukemia
  Optic nerve glioma
  Neurofibromatosis
  Meningioma
  Fibrous dysplasia
  Histiocytosis syndromes
  Metastatic disease
Miscellaneous
  Postirradiation
  Postenucleation
  Trauma
Inflammatory
  Orbital cellulitis
  Orbital abscess
  Orbital pseudotumor
  Trichinosis
Vascular disorders
  Hematoma
  Hemangioma
  Varicosities
  Arteriovenous malformations

In clinical practice, orbital cellulitis is the most frequently encountered orbital disease producing proptosis in childhood. We have diagnosed and treated this condition much more frequently than any other specific orbital entity. With regard to tumors of the orbit (Table 2), dermoid cyst and hemangioma are responsible for 47% to 61% of all orbital tumors in children. When rhabdomyosarcoma and metastatic neuroblastoma are added, these four tumors comprise 60% to 74% of all orbital tumors in childhood. However, in our experience, dermoid cysts have been found to occur more frequently anteriorly, attached to the orbital rim either at the medial or lateral aspect of the superior orbital rim. Only occasionally have these cysts extended into the orbit, and when this has occurred in children the orbital involvement has been minimal.

TABLE 2. Frequencies of various orbital tumors in children: clinical centers (histologic diagnosis)*

Tumor	Series						Total (263)	
	Ingalls		YoussEffi		Iliff and Green			
	Number of cases	Percent	Number of cases	Percent	Number of cases	Percent	Number of cases	Percent
Dermoid cyst	15	29.4	29	46.7	39	26.0	83	31.6
Hemangioma	14	27.4	9	14.5	18	12.0	41	15.2
Rhabdomyosarcoma	4	7.8	2	3.2	16	10.7	22	8.4
Neuroblastoma	3	5.9	6	9.7	2	1.3	11	4.2
Neurofibroma	4	7.8	0	0	6	4.0	10	3.8
Pseudotumor	2	3.9	2	3.2	5	3.3	9	3.4
Glioma of optic nerve	1	2.0	1	1.6	7	4.7	9	3.4
Meningioma	1	2.0	0	0	5	3.3	6	2.3
Lymphangioma	0	0	0	0	6	4.0	6	2.3
Leukemia and lymphoma	3	5.9	0	0	2	1.3	5	1.9
Schwannoma	2	3.9	0	0	3	2.0	5	1.9
Lipoma	0	0	0	0	4	2.7	4	1.5
Microphthalmos with cyst	0	0	0	0	4	2.7	4	1.5
Postoperative granulation tissue	0	0	0	0	4	2.7	4	1.5
Retinoblastoma:								
Extrabulbar extension	—	—	—	—	4	2.7	4	1.5
Orbital recurrence	—	—	—	—	4	2.7	4	1.5
Orbital presentation	—	—	—	—	2	1.3	2	0.8
Teratoma	0	0	0	0	3	2.0	3	1.1
Epithelial or sebaceous cyst	0	0	2	3.2	1	0.7	3	1.1
Prolapsed fat	0	0	0	0	3	2.0	3	1.1
Unexplained proptosis	0	0	3	4.8	0	0	3	1.1
Dermolipoma	0	0	2	3.2	0	0	2	0.8
Fibrous dysplasia	0	0	1	1.6	1	0.7	2	0.8
Organizing hematoma	1	2.0	1	1.6	0	0	2	0.8
Undifferentiated sarcoma	0	0	0	0	2	1.3	2	0.8

Neurosarcoma; sphenoid wing meningioma; ectopic lacrimal gland; thyroid exophthalmos; metastatic embryonal sarcoma; meningoencephalocele, eosinophilic granuloma; mixed tumor of lacrimal gland; leiomyosarcoma; medulloepithelioma; alveolar soft part sarcoma; metastatic astrocytoma; fibrous histiocytoma; myxosarcoma (one of each).

*After Nicholson, D. H., and Green, W. R. Tumors of the eye, lids, and orbit in children. In Harley, R. D., editor: *Pediatric Ophthalmology*, Philadelphia, 1975, W. B. Saunders Co., p. 1,001.

When considering the possible causes of orbital disease, one must consider that any of the many tissues that make up the orbit and its contents can undergo benign or malignant neoplastic change, blood vessels may become altered in their anatomic relationships, neoplastic and inflammatory metastatic disease may find its way to the orbit, the orbit and its contents are subject to a wide variety of direct infections and inflammatory change, and finally, the orbit and its contents may suffer from malformation and malfunction due to faulty development or trauma. When confronted with orbital disease, a logical orderly plan should be carried out in diagnosis.

Since deep orbital contents are difficult to study, even with adequate surgical exposure all necessary indirect evidence should be obtained before surgical intervention. The list of potential orbital diseases is long, and many are relatively uncommon but still significant. The ophthalmologist should consider enlisting the aid of other physicians. For example, the hematologist-oncologist or pediatric surgeon can aid in interpretation of catecholamines, peripheral blood and bone marrow, renal or abdominal masses, vanillymandelic acid (VMA), abdominal palpation, interpretation of intravenous pyelogram, and so on.

Developmental disorders

Orbit growth is stimulated by the presence of a globe, or, in cases of enucleation in infants, by the presence of an implant. Kennedy[23] found a 15% decrease in orbital measurements on x-ray film when no implant was used and of only 8% when an implant was used in a series of patients whose eyes were enucleated between age 1 day and 14 years. The difference in orbital volume may be as much as 50% greater under the same circumstances. The younger the patient in whom an enucleation is done, the smaller will be the orbit. However, clinically significant cosmetic disfigurement is seldom caused by the smaller bony orbit in either a patient who has undergone enucleation or in a unilaterally microphthalmic patient. A smaller palpebral fissure is the most significant factor in the patient with unilateral microphthalmos. In other words, problems caused by the related soft tissue changes are most significant. Patients who have had irradiation following enucleation of one or both eyes for retinoblastoma have a characteristic reduction of bone growth in the midface, including the orbits, that is cosmetically significant.

Shallow orbits occur in Crouzon disease, Apert syndrome, Pfeiffer syndrome, and other craniofacial anomalies. Each is characterized by a significant abnormality of the facial and skull bones and each is transmitted as an autosomal dominant trait with variable expression.

The most extreme forms of craniofacial deformities occur in monsters who are stillborn. Other severe facial deformities including orbital deformities have been treated by a complex surgical procedure that mobilizes and restructures the bones of the midface and orbit. This procedure, described by Tessier,[45] has been associated with complications including cerebral edema, optic atrophy, and hydrocephalus; however, when successful, it can enhance a patient's appearance to the point that he or she has a more realistic chance to function in society. Spontaneous subluxation of the globes is eliminated, and optic atrophy may be prevented by successfully repositioning the orbital walls and midfacial bony structures.

PLATE 9-4

A Crouzon disease in a 4-year-old boy.

B **(1)** Microphthalmos OD; **(2)** microphthalmos with cyst OD in a 6-year-old girl.

C Pfeiffer syndrome: **(1)** facial features; **(2)** syndactyly.

D Midface cleft.

Dermoid cyst

Dermoid cyst is the most common orbital tumor, comprising about one third of all such tumors. However, most dermoid cysts are attached to the orbital rim and are not truly in the orbit if one considers the orbital septum to be attached at the anterior extent of the orbit. These tumors arise from a congenital abnormal retention of ectodermal tissue, usually at a suture line, and they enlarge slowly because of the desquamation of stratified squamous epithelium. The walls of the cyst contain accessory skin structures, including hair follicles and sebaceous glands. About one half of dermoid cysts are attached to the superior orbital rim at the upper outer quadrant, and one quarter are at the nasal aspect of the superior orbital rim. These tumors are firm, round or oval, discrete, and are attached to bone, usually at a suture. They may be removed intact quite easily if care and patience are used by the surgeon. We have seen two dermoid cysts extend into the orbit in children under age 5, but the extension was small and without significant proptosis. When excised completely, dermoid cysts do not recur. About half of all dermoid cysts will become evident by age 12 years. Treatment is complete surgical excision when possible.

Hemangioma

Cavernous hemangiomas occurring in the orbit in infancy and in childhood often but not invariably undergo partial or complete involution. They usually begin as a discoloration of the skin, and in the first few months of life they may undergo rapid enlargement until the lesion stabilizes or begins to involute. After this, roughly 80% of the tumors regress in size, but this process may take months to years. This "involuting hemangioma" as described by Green[16] is most commonly of the capillary variety, with the cavernous type occurring less frequently. Often, individual tumors have both cavernous and capillary components. The majority of this type of hemangioma in childhood occur in the lids and anterior orbit. Proptosis and blepharoptosis are common. When strabismus and blepharoptosis occur, the amblyopia produced may be profound.

Small anterior hemangiomas may be excised successfully. Surgical excision or partial excision, steroids, irradiation, sclerosing solution, and cryotherapy have been used for the treatment of more posterior lesions. Sclerosing solution seems to be of limited effectiveness, since its effects are unpredictable and probably dangerous enough that its use should be discouraged. Transcutaneous cryotherapy is of limited or of no value, but freezing an encapsulated lesion in order to remove it with the cryoprobe seems to be helpful.

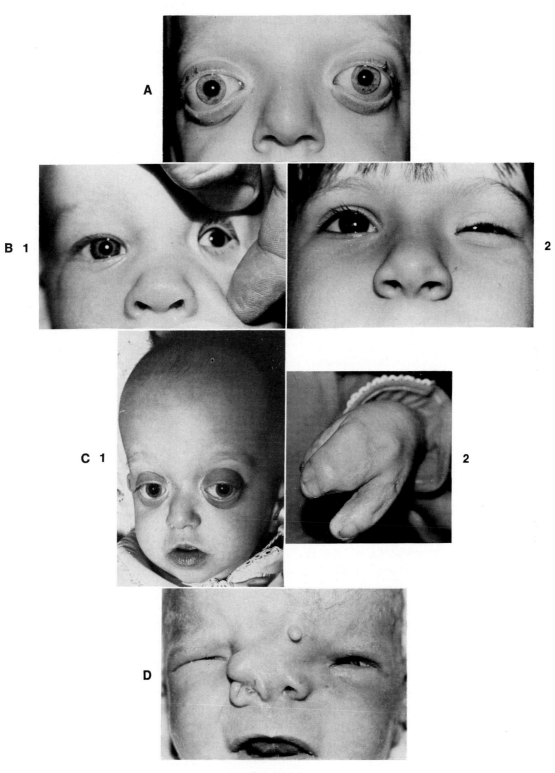

PLATE 9-4

External beam irradiation should be given only in small doses and only when vision is threatened. Higher dosages of irradiation may result in unacceptable scarring and retardation of bone growth as well as the possible later occurrence of neoplastic change in the area.

Radon seeds, which can be applied to the interior of the tumor, must be applied with care, particularly with regard to the expected irradiation level at the lens in the eye. Steroids have been successful in initiating the involutional process in some cases, although a rebound effect has been reported. The dangers of systemic steroids are significant, and their use must be individualized. Surgical excision can be totally successful in some cases or completely impossible in others. Observation over a period of years has proven successful in many cases but not in all or perhaps not in most. Unfortunately there is no way to predict which case will regress spontaneously or which might respond best to a specific treatment modality. Each case must be individualized. Vision must be preserved by recognizing and treating amblyopia.

As children become older, the hemangiomas tend to decrease in size and are somewhat more encapsulated than in early childhood; therefore, they are more amenable to surgical removal when this is required. Hematocysts may occur at any time. Evacuations may be required if the resultant proptosis is severe.

PLATE 9-5

A Hemangioma of the left orbit **(1)** at age 7 weeks; **(2)** 7 months; and **(3)** 6 years. No treatment had been given.

B Hemangioma in an 8-month-old girl **(1)** before and **(2)** 1 month after receiving 400 rads external beam irradiation.

C Untreated hemangioma that has remained essentially unchanged at **(1)** age 5, **(2)** age 6, and **(3)** age 10.

D Dermoid cyst.

Rhabdomyosarcoma

Rhabdomyosarcoma is the most common primary orbital malignancy in childhood, occurring before age 16 in 90% of cases. This tumor is usually first noted as a unilateral proptosis that progresses at a rapid rate in a child between ages 6 and 9 years. The proptosis usually progresses with the eye being pushed down and out. Chemosis and corneal changes leading even to perforation can occur in only a matter of weeks in particularly rapidly growing tumors.

Three cell types are found in orbital rhabdomyosarcoma: embryonal, alveolar, and undifferentiated. Embryonal is the most common cell type found, comprising three fourths of all orbital rhabdomyosarcoma. Aveolar tumors have the poorest prognosis, followed by embryonal and undifferentiated. Metastases to the lungs, brain, and lymph nodes may occur and usually do within 2 years of the onset of the disease.

Diagnosis of rhabdomyosarcoma is by orbital biopsy. Electron microscopy is sometimes necessary for precise diagnosis. In most instances this can be carried out from an anterior approach through the skin just beneath the orbital rim over the site of a palpable mass. Treatment consists of irradiation with a

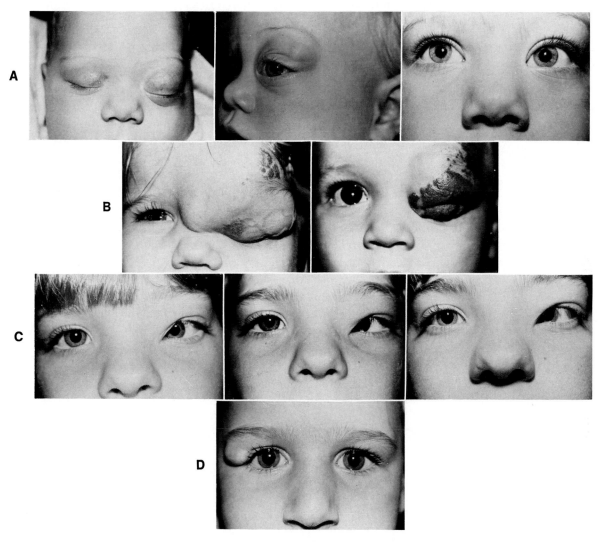

PLATE 9-5

high-voltage external beam. Five thousand rads are given initially with a follow-up treatment of 800 rads. This treatment invariably produces a cataract that may be dealt with surgically if the situation warrants. Chemotherapy consists of vincristine, actinomycin D, and cyclophosphomide. Before the advent of irradiation for rhabdomyosarcoma, exenteration was the treatment of choice. At this time, it is probably not appropriate to completely abandon exenteration, but survival figures indicate that combined irradiation and chemotherapy produce a 3-year survival rate of 75% for rhabdomyosarcoma compared with approximately 33% for older series in which exenteration was employed.

Neuroblastoma

Neuroblastoma derived from sympathetic neural crest tissue is a common malignant neoplasm in childhood that frequently metastasizes to the orbit. Orbital metastasis usually occurs late in the disease, but because the original tumor in the abdomen or along the sympathetic chain may go undetected, the orbital metastasis may be the presenting sign. Proptosis with spontaneous lid ecchymosis in a young child should give rise to suspicion of metastatic neuroblastoma. This condition occurs at a younger age than rhabdomyosarcoma, usually by age 3 years. Diagnosis of neuroblastoma is made by locating the primary tumor by means of intravenous pyelogram, abdominal CT scan, the finding of increased urinary excretion of catacholamine products, and bone marrow studies. X-ray and bone scan of the orbital mass may be helpful in confirming the bone changes and metastatic activity associated with the tumor. If any confusion with rhabdomyosarcoma exists, biopsy may be indicated.

Neuroblastoma is treated with irradiation to single metastases and with chemotherapeutic agents, but the survival rate is less than 10% when orbital metastases are present.

Other orbital diseases

Proptosis in childhood may also be caused by eosinophilic granuloma or the other histiocytosis X (Letterer-Siwe or Hand-Schüller-Christian disease). Although the first is radiosensitive to small doses (a few hundred rads), the other two conditions have a much graver prognosis and are less likely to respond to irradiation.

The most common cause of childhood proptosis in most series is orbital cellulitis. Because of the threat to vision posed by orbital swelling, treatment with appropriate parenteral antibiotics while the patient is hospitalized is usually undertaken. Preseptal cellulitis may mimic true orbital cellulitis but has less serious implications.

PLATE 9-6

A Rhabdomyosarcoma in a 7-year-old girl. Proptosis was first noted approximately 3 weeks before this photograph was taken.

B Proptosis caused by metastatic neuroblastoma.

C Proptosis caused by eosinophilic granuloma.

D Preseptal cellulitis.

E Orbital cellulitis.

232

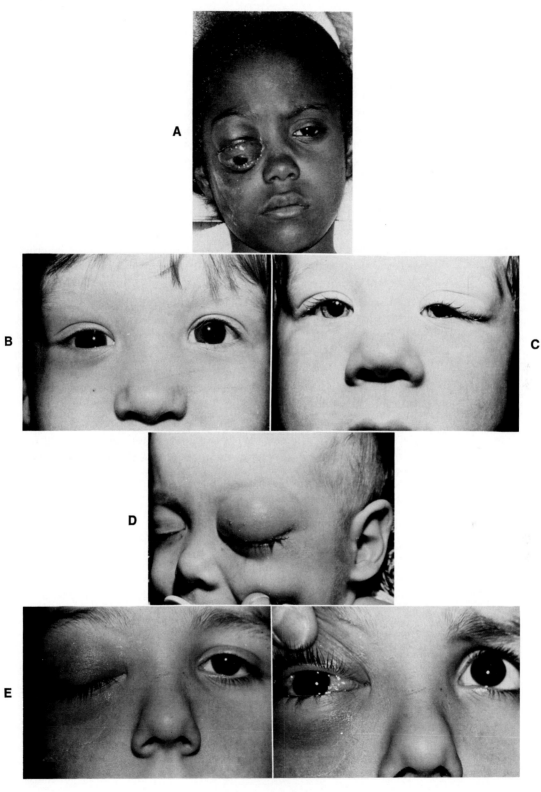

PLATE 9-6

233

SURGERY OF THE ORBIT

In spite of appropriate diagnostic studies of orbital lesions, biopsy or excision is sometimes required. Hemangiomas may be removed completely as may lesions such as dermoid cysts. On the other hand, a biopsy may be required to establish a tissue diagnosis before radiation or chemotherapy. For lesions that require some sort of orbital surgery, two general approaches are taken by the ophthalmologist: a direct approach through skin or conjunctiva over a palpable, anterior lesion or the modified Krönlein lateral orbitotomy. More indirect surgical approaches may be undertaken by the neurosurgeon or the ear, nose, and throat surgeon for tumors that should be approached via the cranial vault or in conjunction with the paranasal sinuses.

PLATE 9-7

A When the anteriorly located lesion can be palpated, a biopsy may be carried out through a skin or conjunctival incision. The lesion is usually located superiorly when this can be done.

B A lateral orbitotomy affords a satisfactory view of the posterior orbit. It is done by first locating the lateral rectus and placing a 4-0 black silk traction suture through the insertion. This provides a handle for adducting the globe, and tug on the suture helps in locating the lateral rectus deep in the orbit. A skin incision begins at the lateral canthus and is carried down to periosteum at the lateral orbital rim. The incision continues laterally for 25 cm through skin and subcutaneous connective tissue.

C The lateral canthal tendon is cut and the orbital rim, which is still covered with periosteum, is exposed upward and downward to points level with the roof and floor of the orbit. At the posterior extent of the incision, temporalis muscle is seen. The orbital rim is cut with a Stryker saw or with a chisel and mallet just below the roof and above the floor of the orbit.

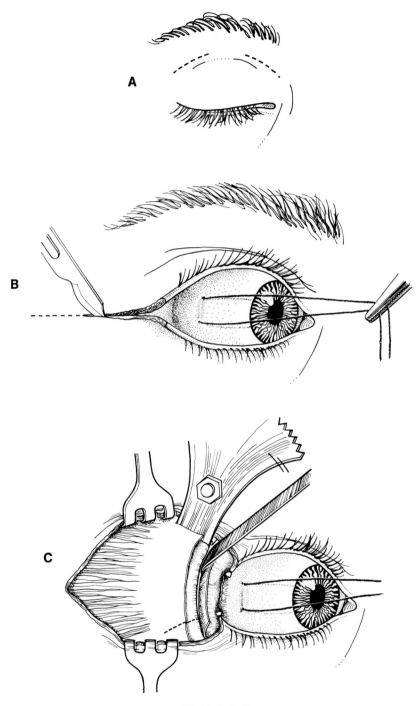

PLATE 9-7

PLATE 9-8

A When cuts have been completed through the lateral orbital rim, the periosteum is incised vertically, and the rim is grasped with a heavy hemostat and fractured laterally, exposing the periorbita.

B The periorbita is incised, exposing the orbital contents.

C Closure is carried out by reapproximation of the periorbita, reattachment of the lateral canthal tendon, closure of deep tissues, and closure of skin.

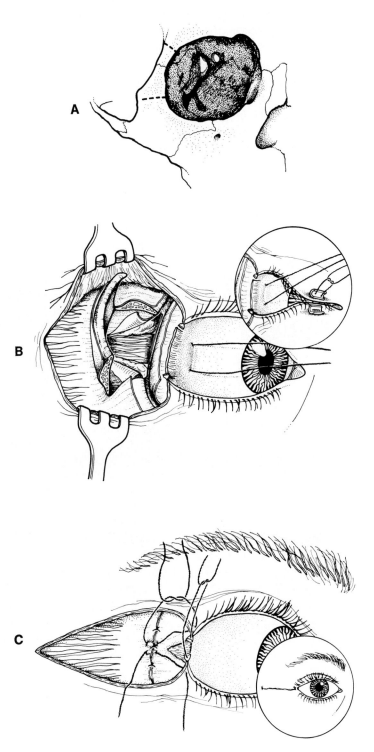

PLATE 9-8

237

PLATE 9-9

A Congenital cystic eye **(1)** at age 1 day; **(2)** excised specimen; **(3)** at age 9 after revision of socket and with prosthesis.*

B Bilateral microphthalmos with cyst.

C Microphthalmos of left eye.

D (1) Soft tissue changes after treatment of retinoblastoma with 10,000 rads. **(2)** Retarded orbital bone growth in another patient 10 years after irradiation treatment in excess of 6,000 rads for retinoblastoma.

———————

*Plate **A**(3) courtesy Alan Putterman, M.D., Chicago.

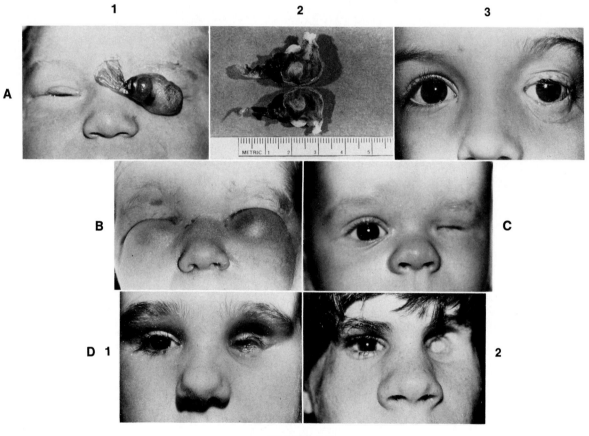

PLATE 9-9

Chapter 10

INFECTIONS, INFLAMMATIONS, AND DEVELOPMENTAL ABNORMALITIES

OPHTHALMIA NEONATORUM AND CONJUNCTIVITIS OF CHILDHOOD

Ophthalmia neonatorum remains a continuing source of concern to the pediatrician and to the ophthalmologist, and its incidence may be increasing. The etiology of ophthalmia neonatorum has changed considerably over the years, and the definition of the term has been broadened to include *all* those infectious disorders of the eye that occur during the first months of life rather than the more narrow definition of gonococcal conjunctivitis.

The infant with ophthalmia neonatorum may develop obvious signs of conjunctivitis within 24 to 48 hours after birth. Most states in the United States still require the administration of 1% silver nitrate solution as a prophylaxis (Credé) against ophthalmia neonatorum. The chemical irritation from this solution is probably responsible for the major portion of inflammatory response "conjunctivitis" during the first 48 hours. This inflammation subsides within a few days.

The next most common cause of ophthalmia neonatorum is hospital-acquired staphylococcal conjunctivitis, the incidence of which ranks next to inclusion conjunctivitis, followed by streptococcal and pneumococcal conjunctivitis, with gonococcal conjunctivitis being relatively uncommon (although its incidence is increasing). Diagnosis in all cases is best established by obtaining gram- and Giemsa-stained conjunctival smears and by doing cultures of conjunctival exudates.

While the time of onset of the conjunctivitis may be a clue as to the etiolog-

239

ic agent, the smear and culture method is the only accurate way to make the precise diagnosis required for appropriate therapy and also is valuable for medicolegal purposes. Sensitivity studies indicate appropriate antiinfective agents.

Conjunctivitis in the older infant and child may originate from many sources, and its duration, severity, and complications may vary widely. Most conjunctivitis in children is self-limiting and may not be brought to the attention of the physician, but it may be epidemic or of such severity as to warrant etiologic investigation and therapy. Complications may be of such severity as to produce corneal ulceration, perforation, and loss of the eye, but the usual goals of identification and treatment are those of shortening the course of the disease and preventing spread to other people. Conjunctivitis may spread from the eye to contiguous structures, or the eye may become involved by a spread of infection from sinuses and adjacent tissue to the orbital tissues. Younger children do not usually complain specifically of conjunctival irritation, but increased discharge from the eyes is apparent to others, crusts or flakes on the lashes are visible, and the lids may be sealed together in the mornings by dried secretions. Conjunctiva is inflamed, and frequent blinking and rubbing of the eyes are evident. Increased tearing is present, and chemosis, edema of the lids, and the presence of preauricular nodes may be apparent.

Closer inspection of the eye may demonstrate follicles in the lower fornix and beneath the upper lid. Papillary hypertrophy and membranes or pseudomembranes may be present. Subconjunctival hemorrhages may be a prominent characteristic. The hyperemia that occurs with conjunctivitis may be mild or severe. Conjunctival hemorrhages may occur with any acute inflammation. Hemorrhagic conjunctivitis, therefore (conjunctivitis marked by the presence of a significant amount of conjunctival hemorrhage) represents a hyperacute inflammatory state and is nonspecific, although organisms typically producing this sequence are *Diplococcus pneumoniae* and the *Haemophilus aegyptius*. Acute hemorrhagic conjunctivitis also is a specific diagnosis of an epidemic viral disease seen most often in Asia and Africa, the virus being related to the polio virus.

The character of the discharge from the eye may be a helpful diagnostic clue. The initial increase in goblet cell secretions due to inflammation produces a mucoid discharge that later becomes mucopurulent as debris is accumulated. Chemosis of the conjunctiva is classically associated with trichinosis infestation but is a nonspecific sign. Papillary hypertrophy also is nonspecific, as are follicles that are quite common in the lower fornix and cul-de-sac of children. Papules can be recognized as a tuft of blood vessels, often with a central vascular core. Follicles, on the other hand, are areas of accumulated lymphoid tissue and, when pathologic, are seen in patients having viral and chlamydial infections. Since follicles in the lower fornix are almost universally present in children, the superior tarsal area must be examined before the presence of follicles can be said to be significant.

Whether a membrane or a pseudomembrane forms depends upon the acute nature of the infection. A disease process that is producing a rapid release of serum and fibrin that coagulates within the epithelial layer produces a true membrane, which when removed will tear the conjunctival surface, leaving a raw, bleeding surface. A slower process, in which the coagulation occurs on the conjunctival surface rather than within the tissues, produces a pseudomembrane that is not incorporated into the epithelium and that does not produce bleeding when removed. Membranous conjunctivitis is typical of epidemic keratoconjunctivitis, streptococcus infections, diphtheria, and other forms of acute purulent conjunctivitis.

Preauricular adenopathy or submandibular adenopathy is characteristic of viral or chlamydial conjunctivitis or Parinaud syndrome (oculoglandular syndrome), the classic syndrome of conjunctivitis and preauricular adenopathy. Very large nodes may be seen with other forms of conjunctivitis, such as syphilis, lymphogranuloma venereum, and tularemia.

Diagnosis and treatment

The initial diagnosis of any type of conjunctivitis is more dependent on a smear for Gram and Giemsa stains, but cultures should be done for definitive diagnosis and for sensitivity studies when indicated. Slides for fluorescent antibodies are diagnostic for types I and II herpes virus and are available in most laboratories. The predominance of polymorphonuclear leukocytes in scrapings from the conjunctival surface suggests the presence of a bacterial or chlamydial infection, except for *Neisseria catarrhalis* and *Moraxella lacunata*, with which Gram and Giemsa stains show mostly mononuclear cells. Mononuclear cells predominate, of course, in viral infections unless significant necrosis occurs, as is seen with membrane formation. Membranes always indicate necrosis, and the presence of polymorphonuclear leukocytes is to be expected. Plasma cells are seen with trachoma; eosinophilia suggest the presence of allergic disease.

The patient presenting with conjunctivitis should have a careful history taken because of the epidemic nature of some forms of the disease. Most are self-limiting and do not require treatment; however, exceptions occur.

If the presence of organisms or an overwhelming number of polymorphonuclear leukocytes on the Gram or Giemsa stain indicate the conjunctivitis to be bacterial, one may begin therapy while awaiting the culture confirmation of that organism and perhaps for the sensitivity studies to suggest more appropriate therapeutic agents. Most epidemic, bacterial conjunctivitis in the northern United States is attributable to *Staphylococcus*, *Streptococcus*, or *Pneumococcus*. These organisms usually are susceptible to the administration of topical bacitracin, erythromycin, or sulfa drugs. The organism usually responsible for this condition in the southern United States is *Haemophilus aegyptius*. This organism responds well to topical treatment with sulfacetamide and erythromycin. It is *not* sensitive to bacitracin. Chloramphenicol may be substituted if required. *H. influenzae* is also sensitive to these agents. Bacterial conjunctivitis due to *Escherichia coli* or *Proteus* and *Pseudomonas* is fortunately rare. The response of these organisms to treatment is less predictable, but most are sensitive to neomycin, chloramphenicol, or sulfa drugs. Gentamycin is more effective for *Proteus* and is often the drug of choice as indicated by sensitivity studies. Chlamydial conjunctivitis is most commonly encountered as inclusion conjunctivitis. Diagnosis is made by conjunctival scraping, Giemsa stain, and the demonstration of inclusions in the epithelial cells. For ophthalmia neonatorum due to inclusion conjunctivitis, topical erythromycin or sulfa is given daily in ointment form for approximately 2 weeks. For parents of infected children or older children with chlamydial infection; tetracycline or erythromycin is given for approximately 3 weeks orally in a daily dose of 1 to 2 g. Trachoma is uncommonly seen in the United States but continues to occur sporadically. Treatment is the same as for inclusion conjunctivitis.

Molluscum contagiosum conjunctivitis is usually unilateral and is diagnosed by noting the presence of a molluscum nodule on or near the lid margin. Treatment is by removal of the lid lesion. Verruca vulgarus causes a chronic papillary conjunctivitis with papillomas that may be present in corresponding positions on the upper and lower lids. It is better to make this diagnosis clinically, treat the lesions with cryotherapy, and avoid incisions because of the risk of spreading the virus through surgical excision.

Parasitic conjunctivitis, although important on a world-wide basis, is seldom seen in the United States. *Phlyctenulosis* is a special type of conjunctivitis due to a delayed hypersensitivity reaction to a variety of organisms. The most common cause is a hypersensitivity reaction due to the presence of *Staphylococcus aureus*. Formerly, the tubercle bacillus was thought to be responsible. This is a self-limiting disorder that begins with a small nodule on the conjunctiva near the limbus either on the corneal or conjunctival side. On the cornea the phlyctenulosis may be accompanied by a leash of blood vessels, which is in itself diagnostic. Associated phlyctenulosis may be found in many patients. Treatment consists of eradicating the associated disease process, which is usually a S. *aureus* infection of the lid margin. If symptoms are extreme, topical steroids are effective.

Viral conjunctivitis is the most common form of conjunctivitis. It is self-limiting, usually lasting only 2 to 4 weeks. It may be accompanied by sore throat when seen as pharyngeal conjunctival fever, in which case it is due to adenovirus type III. Specific diagnosis may be made by serologic tests, but this is usually not necessary. The disease is self-limited, and no specific treatment is required.

INFECTIONS
Corneal infection

Corneal infection may occur as a result of bacterial invasion from a conjunctival focus, by blood-borne metastases, or by direct invasion of disrupted epithelium. Except for herpes simplex keratitis, corneal infection in children is most commonly due to phlyctenular disease or to direct invasions of the epithelium following an injury. Herpes simplex keratitis is readily recognized by the typical appearance of the dendrite. Children with compromised immune systems may develop herpes zoster keratitis, which can be distinguished in most cases by the associated presence of dermatomally distributed skin lesions. Treatment of herpes simplex should consist of debridement of the lesion, patching of the affected eye, and idoxuridine or adenine arabinoside topically if required.

242

PLATE 10-1

A Ophthalmia neonatorum.
B Large chalazion that required excision.
C Staphylococcal blepharitis.
D Chickenpox lesion affecting the cornea.

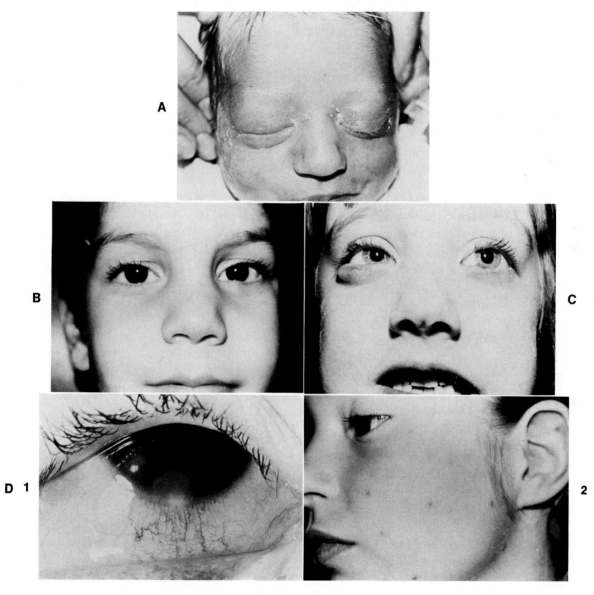

PLATE 10-1

Corneal infection due to bacterial disease, of course, must be treated with antibiotics after appropriate efforts have been made to identify the offending organism. Because of the implications of this type of infection, treatment must be initiated before definitive diagnosis.

Epidemic keratoconjunctivitis may also be seen with sore throat and gastrointestinal symptoms in children. The disease may present as a unilateral conjunctivitis and may be accompanied by pseudomembrane formation. The disease is generally due to adenovirus 8 and may be diagnosed by serologic tests. The presence of subepithelial opacities, developing a week or 10 days after the onset of the conjunctivitis, is characteristic. The opacities may persist for several months and may produce photophobia or reduce vision but eventually disappear. Treatment is nonspecific. Some recommend steroids topically for the suppression of the subepithelial opacities, but others feel that this prolongs the disease.

Acute hemorrhagic conjunctivitis occurs in epidemics, and hemorrhages are generally noted on the upper bulbar conjunctiva. No treatment is available, nor is it required.

Lid infections

Staphylococcal blepharitis is a common cause of the encrustation and discharge seen along the lid margins of infants and children. Often a mild conjunctivitis may be present that is secondary to toxic products from the bacteria. Since the infection is in and around the Meibomian glands and hair follicles, treatment must be directed to these sources rather than to the conjunctival sacs. The primary therapy for this disorder is meticulous lid hygiene and topical antibiotic ointment to the lid margins.

The "collarettes" of staphylococcal blepharitis consist of accumulated secretions that surround the lash and progress further up the shaft as the lash grows. This feature can be helpful in differentiating staphylococcal blepharitis from seborrheic blepharitis. In seborrheic blepharitis the greasy scales and flakes lay on the lashes and are not as closely adherent. Seborrhea of the scalp is always present. Treatment must be directed at the scalp, but weak antiseborrheic shampoos may be used on cotton-tipped applicators to facilitate the cleaning of the lashes.

Hordeola, or styes, result from bacterial infection, usually staphylococcal, of a sebaceous gland. They have rather rapid development and proceed to spontaneous evacuation in a few days. They may be treated with warm compresses and topical antibiotic ointment.

Chalazia result from granulomatous inflammation of the Meibomian glands and often produce a firm, mildly tender mass in the lid (tarsal plate) that persists over many weeks or months. If spontaneous resolution does not occur or if astigmatism and blurred vision are produced, the chalazion should be evacuated. A variety of methods has been suggested, but the most effective and simplest seems to be a vertical incision into the lesion from the conjunctival side, sparing the lid margin. The contents of the lesion can then be evacuated by currettage.

Fungal infections

Fungal infections occur as a result of truama, usually produced by vegetable matter such as a stick or a leaf edge injury to the cornea. They are characterized by extreme discomfort but exhibit less inflammatory reaction than might be expected. A plaque is usually found on the posterior corneal surface. Metastatic fungal disease, frequently *Candida,* may occur in immunosuppressed children.

Specific antifungal agents such as amphotericin B, pimaricin, or flucytosine can be used.

INTRAOCULAR INFLAMMATION

Children are affected with relatively few intraocular inflammatory processes but, unfortunately, when the child's eye becomes involved in such a process the ultimate visual outcome is frequently poor. Viral conditions to be considered with intraocular inflammation include the following:

1. Rubella. The presence of pigmentary retinopathy of the "salt and pepper" type along with cataracts, glaucoma, hearing disorders, and cardiac anomalies is strongly suggestive of rubella infection. When present in the newborn, it is due to the transplacental migration of the virus from the mother's circulation to the fetus. Incomplete aspiration of these cataracts in the first 2 or 3 years of life may produce violent inflammatory response in the eye, and chronic uveitis may persist indefinitely.

2. Herpes simplex. An anterior chamber reaction may occur as a result of epithelial and stromal herpes simplex. Live virus has been recovered from the anterior chamber in the presence of the infection.

3. Subacute sclerosing panencephalitis. The measles virus may produce chronic intraocular inflammation along with retinal and choroidal changes.

4. Cytomegalic inclusion disease. This condition is often congenital but may be acquired by an immunosuppressed child. Retinochoroiditis occurs, which is difficult to distinguish from toxoplasmic retinochoroiditis by appearance. Diagnosis is established by serologic testing or by urinalysis for CMV bodies.

Many other systemic viral infections may produce a chronic uveitis of a nongranulomatous nature.

Bacterial causes of intraocular inflammation in children include virtually the entire spectrum of pathologic and opportunistic organisms. Trauma may introduce organisms of any type into the eye. Metastatic bacterial endophthalmitis occurs frequently with certain disorders such as meningococcemia. This complication may be easily overlooked because of the severe systemic implication of the primary disease. *Hemophilus* appears to be a frequent metastatic organism in children. Hypopyon may occur as a complication of severe corneal inflammation. The heavy exudate in the eye is usually sterile.

Tuberculosis may produce iridocyclitis and choroiditis. Greasy keratic precipitates occur on the cornea. Miliary tuberculosis may produce innumerable foci of infection in the choroid.

Interstitial keratitis and anterior uveitis occur. Chorioretinitis also occurs, usually with marked pigment dispersion and hypertrophy.

Nonspecific intraocular inflammatory disease occurring in children includes:

1. Traumatic iridocyclitis. Pain, miosis, and anterior chamber inflammation occur as a result of trauma to the globe.

2. Endogenous inflammation of unknown causes such as is seen with Still disease and collagen disease, regional enteritis, and ulcerative colitis.

3. Peripheral uveitis (pars planitis) is a disorder of unknown etiology that affects rather selectively the pars plana area. The disorder is characterized by accumulations of white deposits of inflammatory material in the pars plana area, particularly inferiorly. The course of this disease may be a protracted one. The macula may be secondarily affected by cystoid changes, with variable loss of vision.

4. Sympathetic ophthalmia.

Treatment

With any form of intraocular inflammation, treatment may be both symptomatic and specific. Standard treatment programs for the relief of discomfort apply to all forms of inflammation. Cycloplegic agents are effective in relieving discomfort and in reducing the incidence and severity of synechia due to inflammation although in specific cases pupillary mobility may be of equal importance. Long-acting cycloplegic agents might increase the risks of the pupil becoming adherent to the lens or cornea in the dilated position. Patching is generally discouraged except for herpetic and viral disorders unless it is to be for only 24 to 48 hours, as when dealing with a corneal abrasion.

Ice bags and systemic medications for pain relief are helpful in individual cases. Steroids, topically, by local injection, and systemically, are successful in reducing the inflammatory response in many cases. Their potential benefits must be weighed against their potential risks in each case. They cannot be considered specific therapy for any specific ocular inflammation. Other immunosuppressive agents may be helpful in individual, difficult cases.

Specific forms of therapy include those of debridement of the infected epithelial cells of herpetic lesions, patching to adversely affect the viral particles sensitive to temperature elevation, and antiviral agents to interrupt replication of the virus. Specific antibiotics or antifungal agents can be used when sensitivity studies indicate their probable effectiveness.

DEVELOPMENTAL CORNEAL ABNORMALITIES AND DYSTROPHIES

The earliest corneal abnormalities with which the clinician is confronted are developmental abnormalities. Abnormalities of development that involve the cornea include the following disorders in which the cornea is smaller than normal:

1. Anophthalmos. True anophthalmos is rare, but when present includes the absence of the entire globe and extraocular muscles.

2. Cryptophthalmos. The cornea is incorporated into the skin overlying the globe. No palpebral fissure is present. The lids cannot be separated from the cornea surgically.

3. Microphthalmos with cyst. The eye is quite small and maldeveloped,

although a large cystic mass may occupy the orbit. Microphthalmos is generally the correct diagnosis is those cases where anophthalmos is suspected.

4. Nanophthalmos. The eye is structurally sound but is smaller than normal. Glaucoma may develop later. Hyperopia is frequent.

5. Microcornea. The globe is of normal size, but the cornea is smaller than 10.0 mm in horizontal diameter. Glaucoma may develop. Dominant inheritance may be present.

6. Persistent hyperplastic primary vitreous. The involved eye is smaller than the fellow eye. Ciliary processes may be visible through the pupil. The lens may be cataractous. Remnants of the hyaloid system may be present. The condition is generally unilateral.

Congenital conditions with an enlarged cornea include:

1. Megalocornea. The globe is normal in size but the cornea is enlarged, although otherwise normal. The intraocular pressure is normal. No tears are present in the Descemet membrane. This disorder may be inherited in various ways.

2. Keratoglobus. The entire cornea may bulge forward in globular fashion. The intraocular pressure is normal.

3. Buphthalmos. The cornea and anterior segment are grossly enlarged and perhaps distorted with corneal clouding or edema. Horizontal or circumferential tears in the Descemet membrane may be present. The intraocular pressure is elevated.

4. Unilateral high myopia. Myopia of extreme degree may be present at birth. The cornea and globe may be considerably larger than the fellow eye. Tears in the Descemet membrane may be present.

5. Congenital glaucoma. This condition may be unilateral or bilateral. Horizontal or circumferential tears in the Descemet membrane may be present. Corneal edema may be present. The intraocular pressure is increased.

Other developmental abnormalities of the cornea include:

1. Sclerocornea. All or part of the cornea may be opaque and vascularized. The involved cornea may resemble sclera, and scleral vessels may extend into the cornea. Glaucoma may be present.

2. Anomalies of development that affect the anterior chamber in addition to the cornea are:

   a. Axenfeld anomaly, which is characterized by the presence of posterior embryotoxon but normal intraocular pressure.

   b. Axenfeld syndrome, which is Axenfeld anomaly plus elevated intraocular pressure.

   c. Peters anomaly, which is adherence between the anterior lens capsule and the posterior corneal surface. This condition may be developmental or inflammatory. The cornea is cloudy in the area of contact.

   d. Rieger anomaly. The iris stroma is hypoplastic, and pupillary abnormalities such as dyscoria are present. Iris coloboma, ectopia lentis, and glaucoma may be present. Inheritance is autosomal dominant.

3. Dermoids. Limbal dermoids are seen frequently in association with other abnormalities such as coloboma of the eye or lids, mandibular maldevelopment, preauricular appendages, vertebral dysplasia, hearing disorders, and

Duane syndrome. The corneal lesion may produce severe astigmatism and may slowly enlarge in size. Surgical removal leaves an opacified scar in the involved area.

Causes of congenital cloudy corneas include:

1. Tyrosinosis
2. Congenital dystrophy (Schneider, crystalline)
3. Birth trauma
4. Glaucoma
5. Inflammatory conditions (congenital syphilis, rubella)
6. Mesodermal dysgenesis
7. Sclerocornea

Causes of congenital anesthetic corneas include:

1. Extensive corneal disease of any type (for example, ulceration)
2. Herpetic infection
3. Riley-Day syndrome
4. Aplasia of the V nerve nuclei

Causes of congenital folds and tears in the Descemet membrane are:

1. Glaucoma. Tears are usually horizontal.
2. Birth trauma. Tears are often oblique or vertical.
3. High myopia. Horizontal or oblique tears (usually not seen in "pure" high myopia).
4. Syphilis. Circumferential folds (hypertrophied Descemet's).

Mucopolysaccharide disorders affecting the cornea include types IH, IS, II, IV, VI, and VII. All are inherited as autosomal recessive disorders except for MPS II, which is inherited as a sex-linked recessive. All are characterized by abnormal carbohydrate metabolism with sulfates of heparin, dermotin, or keratin appearing in the urine. Severe systemic abnormalities occur in most of these disorders affecting the skeletal, cardiovascular, and central nervous system. Types IH, IS, II (IV), VI, and VII cause cloudy corneas. Types IH, IS, II, and III have associated retinal pigmentary dystrophic changes. Types IH, III, and VII cause mental deficiency.

Amino acid abnormalities that affect the child's cornea include:

1. Cystinosis. The cornea and conjunctiva along with many other tissues are filled with tiny crystals that impart a haze to the entire cornea. Growth and development may be retarded. The disorders may be transmitted as a dominant or as a recessive. Pigmentary retinopathy may be present.

2. Tyrosinosis. Crystalline deposits occur in the cornea. The central cornea may ulcerate and heal with permanent opacity.

3. Lowe syndrome. The cornea may be cloudy, but this is due to the associated glaucoma. Cataract and aminoaciduria along with mental retardation are present. Inheritance is sex-linked recessive.

4. Phenylpyruvic oligophrenia. Corneal opacities occur along with mental retardation, cataracts, and aminoaciduria.

5. Porphyria. Keratomalacia may occur.

Disorders of the lipid metabolism affecting the cornea of children include:

1. Fabry disease. Angiokeratoma corporis diffusum. A whorllike corneal

dystrophy is present in the corneal epithelium, and a posterior, spokelike cataract is present. The trunk areas have many angiokeratomas of the skin.

2. Juvenile xanthogranuloma. Xanthoma lesions of the cornea occur along with iris lesions, which may lead to spontaneous hyphema.

3. Lipid degeneration. An accumulation of lipids may occur in the cornea as a part of any degenerative corneal disease.

Degenerative processes affecting the child's cornea are:

1. Lipid degeneration, which is generally seen as a part of another disease process such as old scars.

2. Band keratopathy. This disorder is frequently seen, usually as a part of a long-standing intraocular inflammatory process. Calcium deposits occur in the Bowman membrane. Hypercalcemic states, exposure, heredity, and idiopathic etiologies have been reported.

3. Terriens degeneration. This peculiar degenerative process often begins in children in their first decade. It is more common in boys and affects the superior corneal periphery. A deepening furrow may lead to extreme thinning and corneal rupture, especially, with minor trauma. Lipid degeneration may be part of the process.

4. Vitamin A deficiency. Keratomalacia is seen along with Bitot spots and xerosis of the conjunctiva and mucous membranes. Night blindness is usually present.

5. Keratoconus.

Corneal distrophies affecting the anterior membrane of the child's eye include:

1. Meesman dystrophy (hereditary epithelial dystrophy). Cystlike spaces occur in the anterior membrane area, generally within the palpebral fissure area. Corneal erosion with irritation may occur. Dominant transmission is the rule.

2. Stocker and Holt hereditary epithelial dystrophy. This disorder is similar to that described by Meesman. It has been reported to be present at birth in some cases. The epithelium is irregular. Serpiginous lines may appear in the deep epithelium.

3. Reis-Bücklers dystrophy. Opacities appear in the superficial Bowman's area or in the deep epithelium. Recurrent corneal erosion with eventual corneal opacification is the rule. Dominant transmission occurs.

Dystrophies affecting the corneal stroma of the child's eye include:

1. Lattice dystrophy. A dominantly inherited disorder characterized by photophobia and irritation. Amyloid is present between the superficial stroma and epithelium, but deposits occur in all levels of the stroma.

2. Granular dystrophy. Discrete opacities appear in the stroma late in the first decade. There is no photophobia or discomfort. Vision usually remains good. Dominant inheritance is the rule.

3. Macular dystrophy. The entire cornea is affected with diffuse deposition of mucopolysaccharide. Photophobia may occur, and symptoms of discomfort and decreased vision may appear early in life. Inheritance is autosomal recessive.

4. Fleck dystrophy. Small opacities that are discrete appear at all levels of the stroma. Vision is rarely affected. Symptoms of photophobia are uncommon but occur. Inheritance is dominant.

5. Crystalline dystrophy. Crystals appear in the central cornea and may be present at birth. Dominant transmission occurs.

Endothelial dystrophies affecting the child's eye include:

1. Deep polymorphous dystrophy. Small vesicles appear in the area of the Descemet membrane. Dominant transmission occurs. Patients are asymptomatic.

2. Congenital hereditary stationary dystrophy. The cornea is cloudy at birth, but the degree of opacification may increase with time. The Descemet membrane is thin, and presumably the associated endothelial inadequacy causes corneal edema. Dominant transmission occurs.

Chapter 11

TRAUMA

Children are particularly subject to ocular trauma because of their size, predilection toward hazardous play activities, and relative lack of judgment. Regardless of the cause of trauma, the overall management of the child's eye does not differ significantly from that of the adult's except when amblyopia is involved, which is a possibility with any child who is injured from birth to 6 or 7 years of age.

LID LACERATIONS

The most frequent and significant injury to the child's lid is laceration, which generally occurs in the upper lid. There are four basic configurations: horizontal, vertical, avulsion, and puncture.

Horizontal lid lacerations

Horizontal lid lacerations should be repaired in anatomic layers; special attention should be given to the levator aponeurosis. If the horizontal laceration is complete, the layers that should be repaired are the conjunctiva, levator aponeurosis, and skin. The orbicularis oculi generally falls into place.

Vertical lid lacerations

Vertical lid lacerations should be repaired also in three layers. Less chance of levator weakness should occur with vertical lacerations than in horizontal. Special attention should be given to the lid margin to make sure that it is everted slightly toward the lid margin to reduce the likelihood of an undesirable lid margin notch.

Repair of lid lacerations. (PLATE 11-1)

A A horizontal lid laceration should be closed in three layers, including conjunctiva, levator aponeurosis, and skin.
B A vertical laceration of the lid should be closed in three layers beginning with the deepest—conjunctiva and tarsus.
C A second layer is closed, approximating the orbicularis oculi muscle.
D Skin is closed and two sutures are placed in the lid margin, one through the gray line and the second anterior to the lashes.

Avulsion of the lid

Avulsion of the lid must be treated on an individual basis, reapproximating tissue edges anatomically as much as possible. The conjunctiva, levator aponeurosis, orbicularis oculi, and skin are identifiable layers that may be sutured. In any type of lid laceration, absorbable sutures should be used when buried and either absorbable or nonabsorbable sutures used for skin closure. With any type of lid laceration that extends toward the medial aspect, the possibility of canalicular damage should be considered. With extensive injury near either canthus, the canthal tendon should be checked and, if necessary, reattached with 4-0 nonabsorbable suture.

Puncture wounds

Puncture wounds of the lid may appear innocuous, but when this type of injury is encountered, the globe should be examined for a penetrating wound. Sharp objects can cause retinal damage and vitreous hemorrhage by passing through the lid (usually the upper) and entering the eye near the superior ora serrata.

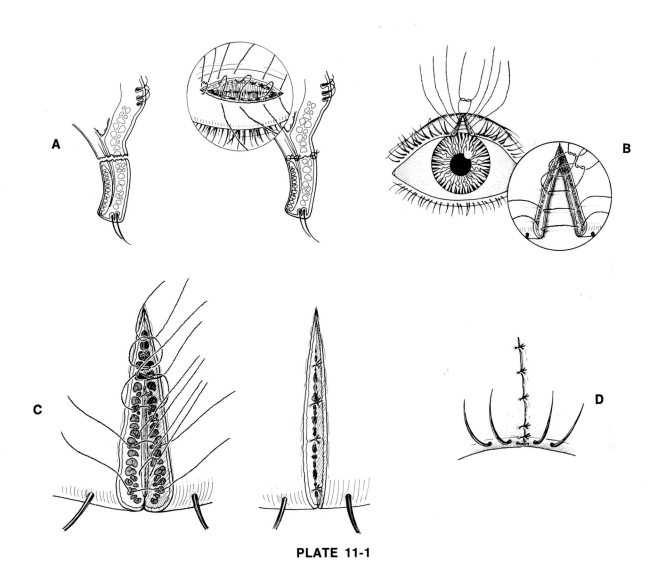

PLATE 11-1

LACRIMAL SYSTEM INJURY

The canaliculi are frequently involved when lacerations occur at the medial aspect of the lids. The upper canaliculus is more frequently involved. When a laceration of either canaliculus is suspected, it should be confirmed or ruled out before proceeding with lid repair. This may be done by dilating the puncta and passing a fine probe through the canaliculus. If the probe can be seen in the wound, the canaliculus has been interrupted. Repair of the canaliculus must then be carried out. For this task, the operating microscope or at least loupe magnification should be used. The distal cut end must be searched for carefully. Retrograde flush of an opaque solution such as steroid suspension through the other punctum is sometimes useful. When the distal cut end is found, a Veirs rod or Silastic tube is placed in it, and the canaliculus is repaired using 10-0 nylon. The stint is left in place for weeks or months. While the lower canaliculus is more important in tear drainage, in some patients up to 50% of the tears are carried by the upper system. Late repair of a severed canaliculus is virtually impossible, and if tearing is sufficient to warrant intervention, a conjunctivodacryocystorhinostomy must be done. We avoid use of a "pigtail" probe on a routine basis because of the potential for damage to the canaliculi caused by stripping of the endothelium or creation of a false passage. However, with careful application, the pigtail probe can be useful in cases in which direct observation of the distal severed end of the canaliculus cannot be accomplished.

Canalicular repair (PLATE 11-2)

A Laceration of the right lower canaliculus.

B Probe through punctum and distal canaliculus can be seen in laceration confirming canalicular laceration.

C *Left,* proximal cut end of canaliculus seen with magnification. *Right,* steroid suspension (or other liquid) injected in upper punctum comes out proximal cut end.

D Canaliculus is repaired with 10-0 nylon interrupted sutures.

E A stint (Veirs rod or Quickert tube) is left in place for 10 day' or 2 weeks.

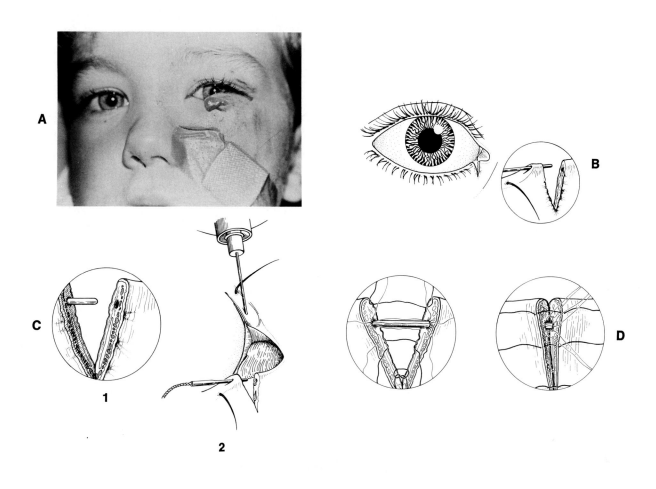

A

B

C

1

2

D

E

PLATE 11-2

255

CORNEAL LACERATION AND BURNS

Corneal laceration in childhood is treated in a manner similar to that in adults. Repair is carried out using magnification and 10-0 nylon sutures. These are left in place for several weeks, and a shield is placed over the eye for several days and may be used for as long as 2 weeks when the patient is sleeping. Children are particularly susceptible to cigarette burns of the cornea, which are inflicted unintentionally by careless adults. This injury is treated with dilatation, topical antibiotics, and a temporary patch. The burn usually heals without a scar.

HYPHEMA

The most common result of serious ocular trauma occurring in childhood is hyphema. Actually, the blood in the anterior chamber is more like the tip of the iceberg. The eye in most cases must receive a rather forceful blow to cause rupture of an iris blood vessel, which produces hyphema. Angle recession can result from this tearing of the iris root (iridodialysis), as can subluxation of the lens, cataract, commotio retinae, or retinal detachment. Any time hyphema occurs, one or all of the panocular sequelae should be considered.

The management of hyphema is varied and controversial. Small hyphemas that occupy 20% or less of the anterior chamber may be managed with bed rest at home (if the family situation is stable) or in the hospital. Patients with larger hyphemas are usually hospitalized with complete bed rest. The injured eye may be patched and a pinhole placed before the fixing eye. Television watching is permitted, but no reading or other activity requiring accommodation should be undertaken. We do not use drops of any kind. Bed rest is continued for 5 to 7 days, after which careful ambulation may resume. If rehemorrhage occurs, it usually does so about the fifth day. After this time, a recurrence of hemorrhage is less likely. The most worrisome acute complication of hyphema is a "black ball" hemorrhage with an acute rise in intraocular pressure. The black ball hemorrhage is removed if pressure remains elevated to 40 mm Hg or more for 24 to 48 hours, although some surgeons remove it immediately. This clot may be removed in a variety of ways, including washing out with fibrinolysin, removal intact with a cryoprobe, and mechanical fragmentation and irrigation. The less instrumentation of the anterior chamber, the better. When a black ball hemorrhage is removed, the complication rate from hyphema increases significantly, the most common complication being cataract. While blood remains in the anterior chamber, increased intraocular pressure can cause blood staining of the corneal stroma. This blood staining is present as a green or brown hue with a lucid ring just inside the limbus. When intraocular pressure is stabilized, the blood stain decreases gradually from the periphery. Resolution is complete in most cases but may require many months.

BLOWOUT FRACTURE

Blowout fracture of the orbit does occur in children; the management is similar to that of the adult. If a large fracture is present, it is repaired with a plate covering the floor deficit after the initial hemorrhage and edema have subsided. With smaller fractures, the patient is followed, and if he improves, surgery is delayed for 10 days. At that time patients with marked restriction and definite x-ray evidence of fractures on tomograms are treated surgically. In a patient with few or no symptoms, surgery is deferred indefinitely.

PLATE 11-3

A **(1)** Blood staining of the left cornea after a black ball hyphema. **(2)** Blood staining of the cornea clearing from the periphery.
B Iridodialysis following blunt trauma.
C Perforation of the globe that occurred as a result of trauma to the upper lid.
D **(1)** Appearance of spectacles after being hit with a BB at close range. **(2)** Iris prolapse from glass fragment that entered the eye. **(3)** Closeup of **(2)**.

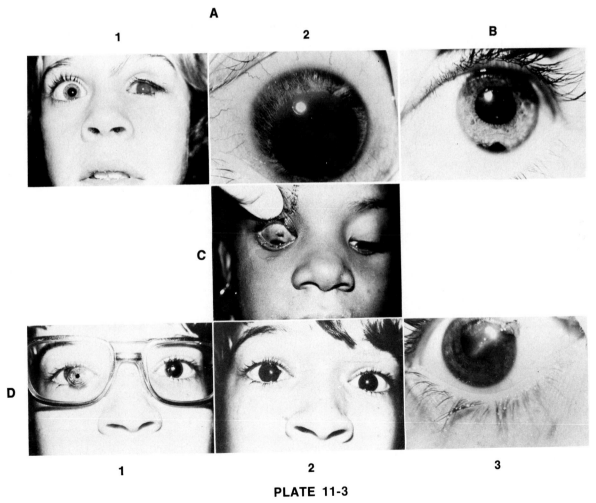

PLATE 11-3

EXTRAOCULAR MUSCLE LACERATION

A rare ocular injury is laceration of an extraocular muscle, most commonly the inferior rectus. The medial rectus is the next most commonly injured. The mechanism of injury is a shearing force causing transection of a rectus muscle just behind the insertion. Since attachments to the intermuscular membrane are intact, the muscle does not retract in the orbit and can usually be found at surgery without much difficulty. Repair of a lacerated muscle is carried out with direct reapproximation and is usually successful. The superior oblique tendon may be transected by an injury such as from a store display hook or a sharp, pointed tool. Retraction of the lower lid on attempted downgaze but without depression of the globe is a tell-tale sign of inferior rectus laceration.

PLATE 11-4

A Avulsion of the left upper and lower lid by a German shepherd. **(1)** Before and **(2)** 4 years after three-stage repair.

B Fracture of the roof of the orbit in a 6-month-old infant.

C Blowout fracture of the orbital left floor causing limited upgaze because of entrapment of the inferior rectus muscle.

D (1) Hypertropia caused by laceration of the left inferior rectus muscle. **(2)** Retraction of left lower lid on attempted downgaze. **(3)** After repair, motility is normal.

258

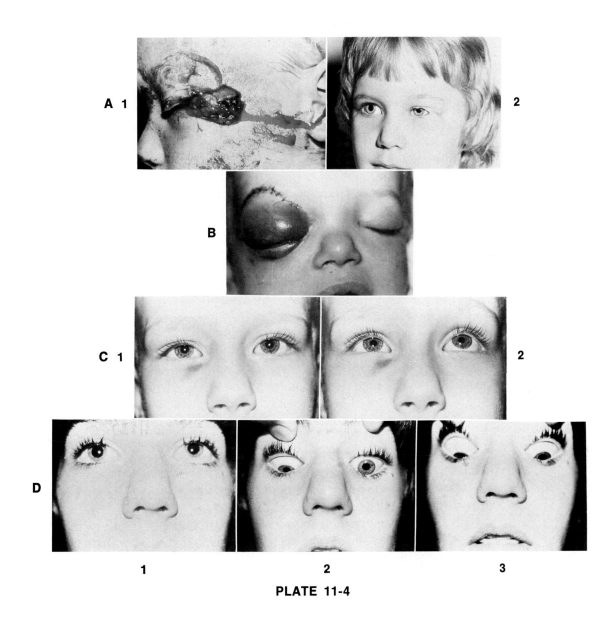

PLATE 11-4

RETINAL INJURIES

Blunt trauma to the globe can cause retinal dialysis or, if the injury is penetrating, a retinal hole may be produced. The usual retinal repair techniques are carried out. Of course, with younger children study of the retina is more difficult and may require an examination with the child under anesthesia.

Hemorrhages in the vitreous usually resolve in children after many months. If a vitreous opacity persists after hemorrhage and especially if it occurs in a child who is young enough to develop amblyopia, vitrectomy may be done.

Penetrating ocular injuries from a pellet or BB gun are usually severe. An ordinary BB gun must be fired from close range to cause penetration. When fired from farther than a few yards, the BB usually does no more than penetrate conjunctiva but may cause contusion of the globe, hyphema, retinal dialysis, or commotio retinae. Double perforations from pellets usually preclude useful vision, but occasionally patients survive repair with some useful sight. Low-velocity missiles are more likely to carry organisms that can lead to endophthalmitis. Iron-containing foreign bodies from such missiles can cause siderosis. Wood or other organic material in the eye can lead to marked inflammatory reaction and fungal infection.

Sympathetic uveitis can occur after an ocular injury associated with prolapse of uveal tissue. The decision to enucleate an eye that has no hope of useful vision should be made promptly and surgery carried out within 10 to 14 days after the injury if the presence of sympathetic uveitis has been ruled out. Contrary to beliefs held by some, sympathetic uveitis can occur in a patient whose exciting eye has had endophthalmitis. Once sympathetic uveitis has started, removal of the exciting eye has no beneficial effect on the inflammatory process. Our usual practice is to carry out primary repair in most severely injured eyes and do an enucleation later if needed as a scheduled procedure after adequate discussion with the family.

Enucleation technique (PLATE 11-5)

A A 360° peritomy is carried out, exposing the rectus muscles.

B Each rectus muscle is severed from the globe. The medial rectus stump is left 4 mm. The superior and inferior oblique muscles may be hooked and severed also at this time.

C Heavy, curved enucleation scissors are placed along the globe *medially* to straddle the optic nerve that is cut. The eye is stabilized by means of an Allis clamp on the medial rectus stump.

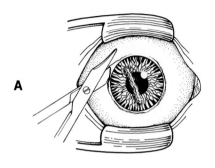

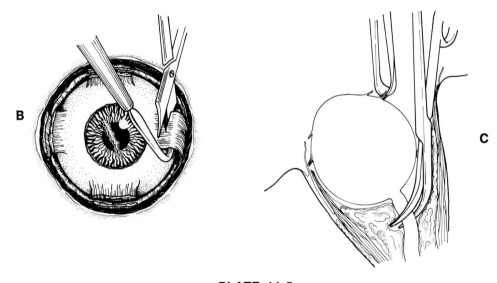

PLATE 11-5

PLATE 11-6

A A silicone implant of appropriate size (12 to 20 mm in diameter) is placed in the muscle cone after pressure has been applied for 5 minutes *by the clock* on the severed central retinal artery and vein; loose gauze can be used to pack the cavity.

B The muscles are joined with a 5-0 synthetic absorbable suture and are closed in a purse string manner. A bite is taken in each muscle and in the intermuscular septum between the muscles.

C The conjunctiva is closed with 5-0 synthetic absorbable suture.

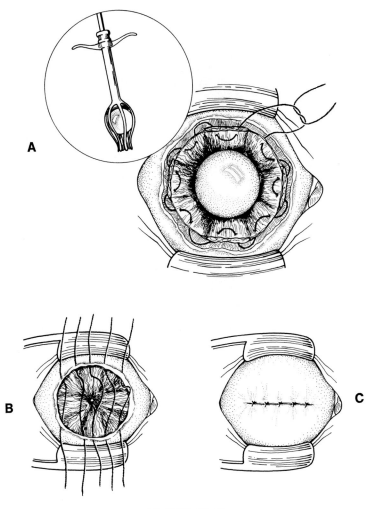

PLATE 11-6

LENS INJURY

The lens may be injured, causing cataract, subluxation or dislocation (see Chapter 4).

PLATE 11-7

Superior subluxation of the lens after blunt trauma.

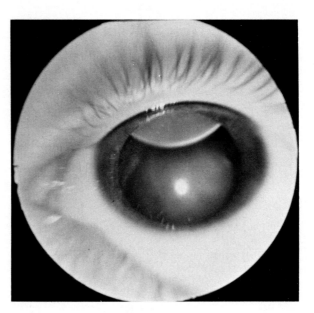

PLATE 11-7

Chapter 12

GENETICS

The blueprint for human development is made up of 23 paired chromosomes, with one chromosome from each pair coming from the mother and the other from the father. These paired chromosomes are found in all cells of the body except the sperm of the male and the ovum of the female, each of which contain 23 unpaired chromosomes. Twenty-two of these chromosome pairs are called autosomes, and they carry the hereditary pattern that determines the inborn or genetic characteristics of the individual. The twenty-third chromosome pair dictates the individual's sex as well as certain other physical characteristics. The mother, by means of the ovum, contributes an X chromosome and the father, by means of the sperm, contributes either an X or a Y chromosome. An offspring whose twenty-third chromosome pair is XX is a female, and the offspring whose twenty-third chromosome pair is XY is a male.

A large number of genetically induced conditions affect the eye directly or indirectly. Some knowledge of the basic principles of genetics is essential for the pediatric ophthalmologist, since this knowledge must be called upon in patient management on an almost daily basis.

Three factors must be dealt with when considering genetics in a clinical setting: (1) Recognition of a disease or condition in an individual (propositus) and determination of other similarly affected blood relatives (pedigree); (2) obtaining appropriate laboratory studies when indicated to confirm the diagnosis of a hereditary disease (as for Tay-Sachs, albinism, Best disease, and so on); (3) knowledge of the method of inheritance for various diseases and use of this information to carry out treatment and to inform and advise the patient.

There are just a few basic patterns for inheritance, and these are basically straight forward. There are also a number of modifying factors that must be understood. Definitions of the more useful genetic terms are:

gene collection of chromosomes that carries the hereditary pattern.
genotype the genetic make-up of the individual.
phenotype the physical makeup of the individual; determined by the genotype but may be modified by the environment.
phenocopy clinical picture resembling a genetically induced condition but produced by the environment and genetically different.
dominant the trait is expressed when one gene of the pair carries it.
recessive the trait is not expressed unless both genes of a pair carry it.
sex-linked trait determined by gene carried on sex chromosome.
regular dominance trait always expressed
irregular dominance trait not always expressed even though the responsible gene is present.
expressivity extent to which gene shows effect.
penetrance frequency of expression.
skipped generation normal phenotype, abnormal genotype.
pleiotropic gene gene with multiple effects.
forme fruste attenuated expression.
multifactorial inheritance characteristics produced by polygenic factors with no sharp distinction between normal and abnormal phenotypes.

PLATE 12-1

Basic inheritance and sex determination. Possible combinations of genes from a male and female parent are shown. The solid round figure demonstrates the X chromosome, and the solid oval figure the Y chromosome. Each of these germ cells contains only 23 chromosomes, but they combine in the offspring to form somatic cells in the offspring that contain 23 *paired* chromosomes. Half the offspring will possess two X chromosomes and be girls; half will contain an X and a Y chromosome and be boys. Each offspring can repeat the cycle with all of the girls' ova containing an X chromosome and half of the sperm cells of the boys containing an X chromosome and the other half a Y chromosome.

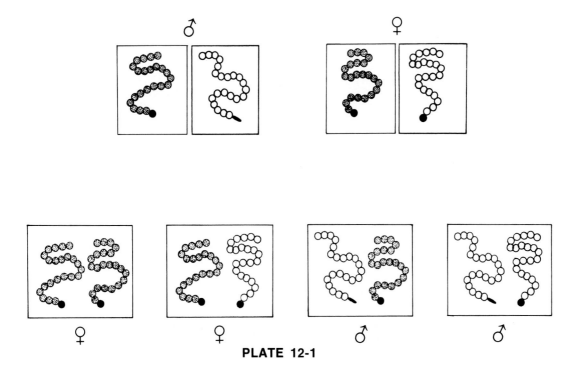

PLATE 12-1

PLATE 12-2

Dominant inheritance. The male parent may have a gene that dictates a dominant trait for a normal characteristic such as brown eyes or for a pathologic condition such as retinoblastoma. He passes this on to his offspring, so that statistically 50% of his offspring (regardless of sex) will have the gene, and since the gene is dominant, they will express the characteristic and pass it on. Although this percentage figure is often quoted, a more accurate statement is that *each* offspring will have a 50% chance of having the gene, and, depending on penetrance, expressing the characteristic.

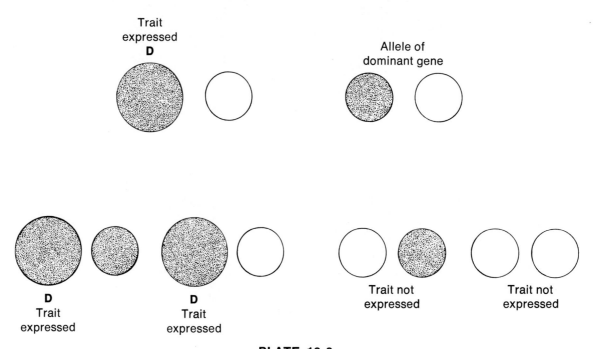

PLATE 12-2

PLATE 12-3

Autosomal dominant inheritance. Both parents carry a dominant gene for the same trait or characteristic. One child will be homozygous for the trait and express it, two children will be heterozygous and express the trait, and one child will be homozygous without the trait. If a parent is homozygous for a dominant characteristic, all children will be heterozygous for the trait and, since it is dominant, will express the characteristic.

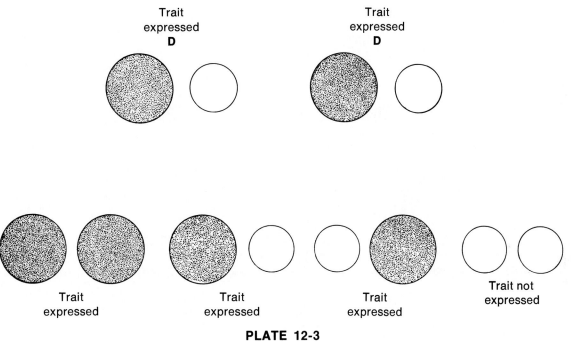

PLATE 12-3

PLATE 12-4

Recessive inheritance. The father passes along a recessive gene to half of his offspring (regardless of sex), who are carriers, but since the gene is recessive, it is not expressed in the presence of a normal allele (gene occupying the same position on the paired set of chromosomes). In some instances the recessive carrier state can be determined by physical appearance or laboratory tests.

Trait not
expressed
(carrier)

r

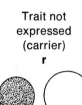

Allele of
recessive gene

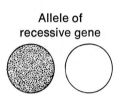

Trait
not expressed
(carrier)

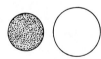

Trait
not expressed
(carrier)

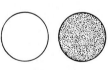

Trait not
expressed

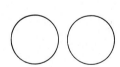

Trait not
expressed

PLATE 12-4

270

PLATE 12-5

Recessive inheritance with expression. Both the male and female parent are carriers of a recessive gene without expression. One offspring will be homozygous for the recessive trait and will express it. Such an example is blue eyes or congenital high myopia. Half the offspring will be carriers, and one fourth will be normal.

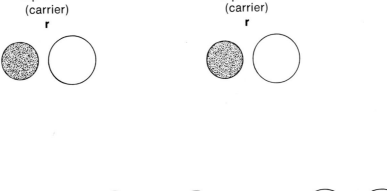

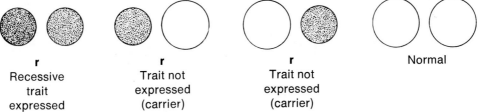

PLATE 12-5

PLATE 12-6

Sex-linked inheritance. The mother carries a recessive trait on the X chromosome. She will pass it along to one daughter who is a carrier and one son who is affected because the Y chromosome is deficient in chromatin and is unable to counteract the recessive trait. Another son will be normal. In other words, one half the sons will be affected, and one half the daughters will be carriers. Ocular albinism is an example of a sex-linked recessive characteristic. Offspring who are homozygous for a sex-linked disease are often stillborn. There are rare examples of sex-linked dominant traits. Hairy ears is the only known trait carried on the Y chromosome.

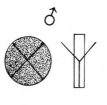
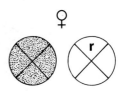

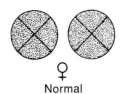
Normal

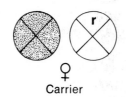
Carrier

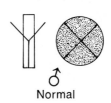
Normal

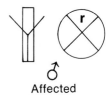
Affected

PLATE 12-6

Chromosomes may undergo aberrations in the form of an addition (trisomy), a totally missing chromosome, or structural abnormalities (deletion, rings, translocation). These occur in 0.5% of live births and in from 20% to 70% of stillborns. Chromosomes are studied by suspending mitosis in leukocytes and separating and then matching chromosomes according to a structural classification. Characteristic karyotypes were first found in Turner, Klinefelter, and Down syndromes. Since then other chromosomal diseases have been studied. The technique is to find a disorder and then do karyotyping in an attempt to find a recurring chromosomal anomaly. In addition to constant chromosomal aberration, mosaicism may exist, in which some cells are normal and others contain abnormal X chromatic material.

Some of the more common diseases that are associated with chromosomal aberrations and that occur sporadically are cri du chat (partial deletion of short arm of chromosome 5), Down syndrome (trisomy 21), Turner syndrome (45X), and Klinefelter syndrome (XXY, XXXY, XXXXY).

Some of the more commonly occurring hereditary ocular diseases and their usual mode of inheritance are the following:

Condition	Mode of inheritance
Achromatopsia	Autosomal recessive
Apert syndrome	Autosomal dominant
Albinism	
Complete (universal)	Autosomal recessive
Incomplete (universal)	Autosomal recessive
Ocular	Sex-linked recessive (or autosomal recessive)
Amish (yellow mutant)	Autosomal recessive
Aniridia	Autosomal dominant or sporadic
Conradi disease	Autosomal recessive
Cornelia de Lange syndrome	Unknown
Crouzon disease	Autosomal dominant
Cystinosis (Fanconi syndrome)	Autosomal recessive
Ehlers-Danlos syndrome	Autosomal dominant
Fabry disease	Sex-linked recessive
Freeman-Sheldon (whistling face) syndrome	Autosomal dominant
Galactokinase deficiency	Autosomal recessive
Galactosemia	Autosomal recessive
Gaucher disease	Autosomal recessive
Goldenhar syndrome (oculoauriculovertebral dysplasia)	Unknown
Hallermann-Streiff syndrome	Autosomal dominant?
Phakomatoses	Autosomal dominant or ?
Homocystinuria	Autosomal recessive
Hyperlysinemia	Autosomal recessive
Incontinentia pigmenti (Bloch-Sylzberger syndrome)	X dominant or intermediate

273

Condition	Mode of inheritance
Kearns-Sayre syndrome (external ophthalmoplegia pigmentary degeneration and cardiomyopathy)	Autosomal dominant
Laurence-Biedl syndrome	Autosomal recessive
Leber congenital amaurosis	Autosomal recessive +
Leber hereditary optic atrophy	Sex-linked or autosomal recessive
Lowe syndrome (oculocerebralrenal)	Sex-linked recessive
Marfan syndrome	Autosomal dominant
Möbius syndrome	Autosomal dominant?
Mucopolysaccharidoses (Hunter syndrome)	Autosomal recessive
	Sex-linked recessive
Niemann Pick disease	Autosomal recessive
Norrie disease	Sex-linked recessive
Peters anomaly	Autosomal recessive
Refsum syndrome	Autosomal recessive
Retinitis pigmentosa	Autosomal dominant
	Autosomal recessive
	Sex-linked recessive
Reiger syndrome	Autosomal dominant
Riley-Day syndrome (familial dysautonomia)	Autosomal recessive
Rubinstein-Taybi syndrome	Unknown
Stickler disease	Autosomal dominant
Sulfite oxidase deficiency	Autosomal recessive
Treacher-Collins syndrome mandibulofacial dysostosis; Franceschetti syndrome)	Autosomal dominant
Usher syndrome	Autosomal recessive
Waardenburg syndrome	Autosomal dominant
	Variable expression
Weill-Marchesani syndrome	Autosomal recessive or dominant
Wildervanck syndrome	Dominant?

Chapter 13

ANESTHESIA

General anesthesia may be given safely to a child of *any age* provided the child is healthy and that the anesthesiologist is competent. This means that in a well infant, surgery, elective or otherwise, can be done without concern for the added "risk" of anesthesia imposed by the age of the patient. If a systemic abnormality such as a cardiac or pulmonary defect is present in a child, the risk of anesthesia increases proportionally to the infant's condition, and the decision to perform surgery with general anesthesia must be made weighing the possible harm that could occur from the condition going untreated and the risk of anesthetizing the child. In a clinical situation, most nonelective ocular surgery in very young infants is done for congenital cataract or congenital glaucoma. Because of concern for the child's developing amblyopia, cataract surgery has been done in the first week of life. Glaucoma surgery is done in the first few months of life. We have done surgery on a week-old infant with impending corneal perforation (conjunctival flap) and have removed a congenital cystic eye from a child at 3 days of age, but these are extreme circumstances.

Strabismus surgery comprises the majority of elective surgical procedures done in the infant. It is our policy to perform surgery for congenital esotropia as early as an adequate diagnosis can be made. This is usually between ages 6 and 12 months.

Preoperative physical examination and routine laboratory tests are done the day before surgery with emphasis on study of the heart, lungs, throat, and ears. The temperature is determined and a urinalysis and complete blood count are obtained (white blood cell count with differential cell count, hemoglobin, and hematocrit). The acceptable values for these tests are usually set by the anesthesiologist, who is always consulted if any question arises regarding the suitability of a child for anesthesia and who examines each patient before administering the anesthetic—usually the night before surgery is to be done.

Children are placed npo (nil per os) 6 hours before surgery. Surgery on younger children is performed first on the operating schedule, which begins at 8:00 AM. Preoperative medication should be kept to a minimum. Some anesthesiologists give none; others give atropine orally with or without a narcotic. Narcotics should ordinarily be avoided because pain is not a usual occurrence after eye surgery and because they contribute to postoperative vomiting. The most important preoperative "medicine" is reassurance for the child old enough to respond to his or her surroundings. Children who have been treated recently with phospholine iodide for glaucoma or strabismus should have blood pseudocholinesterase levels drawn and, if necessary, succinylcholine should be withheld before intubation. Ordinarily, surgery may be done safely if the child has had no phospholine iodide for 6 weeks. If the history provides any reason for concern about hyperthermia, blood levels of creatine phosphokinase (CPK) are determined. A family history of abnormal CPK levels should make the surgeon and anesthesiologist evaluate critically the indication for surgery and should make temperature monitoring mandatory.

The child who is to have surgery should have inhalation anesthesia maintained through an endotracheal tube. This tube allows access to the patient's airway and provides a valuable margin of safety. An intravenous infusion with dextrose 5% and water should be established to provide hydration and to provide means of administering medication if needed. The induction technique and the anesthetic agents used are the choice of the anesthesiologist. Usually, older children have an IV started initially and are given thiopental sodium (Sodium Pentothal) by this route, followed by inhalation of halothane (Fluothane) through a mask. When the child is relaxed, succinylcholine is given to produce muscular relaxation, and the endotracheal tube is placed and anchored. Infants and young children are given halothane via mask for induction initially, and an IV is started later. Fortunately, children are generally amnesic for memory of the mask.

When the child is asleep, a monitor system is established including constant cathode tube display ECG, audible and digital display pulse rate, and digital display temperature. In addition, the anesthesiologist constantly monitors the heart beat and respirations with a precordial stethoscope. A Doppler unit may be of assistance for monitoring the pulse and blood pressure. The surgeon participates in monitoring the child's vital functions by observation of the display, which is on a large console at the end of the operating table.

The most frequent intraoperation problem that we encounter is manifestation of the oculocardiac reflex. This reflex produces a dramatic bradycardia in some children when traction is exerted on the extraocular muscles. For example, the heart rate may go from 120 to 70 in 2 seconds in a sensitive patient when the muscle is engaged with a muscle hook and the eye is rotated. With audible and visual monitoring, the surgeon and anesthesiologist should make the diagnosis at the same time. Treatment of bradycardia from ocular stimulation is initiated by removing all pressure on the muscle. When normal pulse has resumed (usually in a few seconds), a careful tug should be applied to the muscle. Often, the reflex recurs but is less severe. In most cases, the oculocardiac reflex seems to "wear out," and surgery can be resumed. In a few cases it persists. When this occurs, the anesthesiologist may

276

give intravenous atropine and surgery can resume. Because intravenous atropine given in this situation increases the likelihood of arrhythmia, some anesthesiologists prefer to delay in giving the drug. Significant cardiac arrythmias occur rarely in children.

At the conclusion of surgery, it is a good practice to have at least one member of the surgery team remain with the child until he or she reaches the recovery room. Occasionally a child will develop laryngospasm in this period and the anesthesiologist may need assistance while counteracting the spasm.

Unfortunately, children who undergo ocular surgery, particularly strabismus surgery, have a high incidence of postoperative nausea and vomiting. This usually occurs only on the afternoon of surgery and the children are usually comfortable and eating well the next day. It is the contention of the anesthesiologist that the effects of eye surgery cause the vomiting; others (the surgeons) think preoperative narcotic medication may contribute significantly to postoperative vomiting.

Children are allowed to go home the afternoon or evening of surgery or by the next morning. Outpatient surgery with general anesthesia is reserved for patients who live or remain near the hospital (within 40 miles) so that they may be returned to the hospital and admitted if the need should arise.

Outpatient pediatric anesthesia examinations are done using halothane delivered with a mask. These patients are asked to come to the examining area the morning of the examination, the temperature is checked, and the heart and lungs are examined. Simple examination procedures including retinal examination with scleral depression, gonioscopy, intraocular pressure check, retinal photography, retinoscopy, suture removal, and so on are done with halothane delivered through a mask. If lacrimal probing is done, an endotracheal tube is put in place because of concern over possible aspiration of irrigation fluids. We rarely use ketamine dissociative anesthesia because of the long recovery period, but some find it useful, particularly for intraocular pressure examinations.

We virtually have abandoned the use of sedation in an office setting. Most examinations can be done in the office without sedation if enough patience is exercised. Those examinations that require sedation or anesthesia are important enough in our opinion to justify help of an anesthesiologist and are done in a hospital setting.

PLATE 13-1

A Anesthetized patient. **(1)** Endotracheal tube. **(2)** Esophageal stethoscope. **(3)** Nasal temperature probe. **(4)** ECG lead. **(5)** Blood pressure cuff. **(6)** Heating pad. **(7)** Intravenous infusion and Doppler lead are present but not shown in illustration.

B Doppler unit for audible pulse monitoring.

C Monitor with ECG display and digital display of pulse and temperature as viewed by the surgeon.

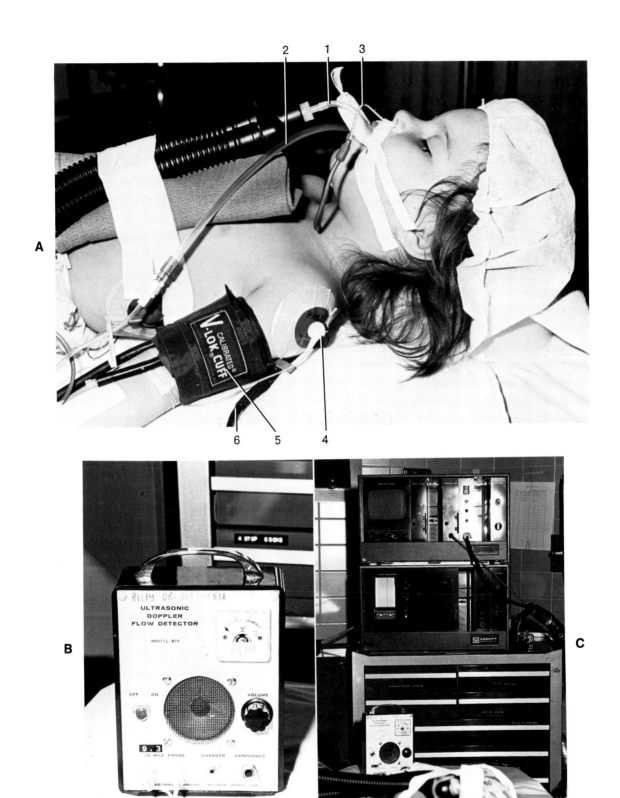

PLATE 13-1

Chapter 14

DYSLEXIA

The problems of learning disability, academic failure, and even delinquent behavior have been thought by some to be due to nonspecific and/or perceptual dysfunction. In the area of academic failure, dyslexia is a term that has become popular as a "socially acceptable" reason for school difficulties in certain children. Because the eyes are used for reading, the ophthalmologist frequently is called upon to answer questions about dyslexia and is asked to examine children and even adults who are thought to have it. The usual setting for the eye examination of the suspected dyslexic patient includes a distraught parent (usually the mother) and a downtrodden but sometimes hyperactive patient (usually a boy). In our experience, the more severe the learning and/or reading difficulty, the earlier the child is seen, but on the average, in the absence of a positive family history, suspected dyslexia patients are seen by grade 3.

The true dyslexic child, that is, the patient with primary specific dyslexia, is not always readily differentiated from the intellectually deprived secondary dyslexic or slow (low IQ) retarded child or endogenous dyslexic. Each does poorly in school and may have behavioral problems, but the problems occur for different reasons. It is very difficult to establish reliable data for academic failures because of vague definitions and because of the wide variety of reasons for this problem. It is a mathematical reality that 50% of all students are below average, and when an individual who is below average happens to reside in a family that expects above average performance, a problem exists.

DEFINITION

Dyslexia simply means difficulty with reading. The term is nonspecific, saying nothing about the cause of this difficulty with reading and implies no etiology. The term has a scientific ring and has become a part of our jargon. Unfortunately, the term has been used by many to describe a diverse group of loosely related academic failures.

Exogenous dyslexia (reading retardation)

The intellectually deprived child may have any level of basic intelligence or IQ but lacks stimulation or specific experience. A child who is reared in a home in which language, either written or spoken, is poorly developed and who attends a crowded classroom supervised by a teacher who may be indifferent or forced to be a disciplinarian runs a very high risk of being a poor reader and an academic underachiever. These patients have been labeled by some as having exogenous dyslexia. This may be a useful term, but it may also serve to create confusion regarding true dyslexia. For example, it would not seem appropriate to label a person dysgraphic for not being able to write if he or she had never been taught to write and never been exposed to writing in a meaningful way. Likewise, it is illogical to label a person dyslexic if he or she has never been taught to read. Because these patients very often come from a deprived background, they are the least likely of all so-called dyslexic patients to be seen by the ophthalmologist. However, these patients do need an advocate, and if they are recognized, appropriate educational diagnostic testing should be carried out, and proper teaching methods should be instituted. These patients should have performance IQ tests done and should be placed in an academic setting that would be most appropriate to their needs. Given the proper opportunity, these people should be able to function up to the expected level of their intelligence. A better term for this condition would be exogenous reading retardation.

Endogenous dyslexia

Some children simply lack the intelligence to become good readers or good students. This lack may be congenital or due to acquired disease or injury. These children have low IQs and are usually diagnosed fairly early in their school careers. This type of "dyslexic" patient should have realistic goals set and should be given the proper academic support to reach these goals.

Primary, specific developmental dyslexia (true dyslexia)

Patients with true specific developmental dyslexia are unable to read at the level that would be expected from their home background, educational opportunities, and their intelligence as measured by performance IQ or nonverbal (written language) methods. In the absence of a positive family history, the child with specific dyslexia may begin to show signs of difficulty as early as the first grade and most certainly will be suspected of having a significant reading difficulty by the third grade. Anyone dealing with the dyslexic or potentially dyslexic child should know that dyslexia is not an all or none condition. Many successful people are minimally dyslexic, with the only manifesta-

282

tion of their difficulty being poor spelling or handwriting, along with slow reading and an inability to read aloud accurately. It would seem that the worst job for a dyslexic individual would be that of a proofreader. Since the dyslexic is a poor speller and a poor decoder, he or she would be expected to have an extremely difficult time finding other's mistakes. This was pointed out by Critchley,[3] who is testing a large number of dyslexic individuals found that they were unable to notice the word "slow" misspelled as "solw" when it appeared in context. Also, these people were unable to detect the error in the spelling of "hospital" when it was spelled "hosiptal." Although having difficulty with reading, handwriting, and spelling, such an individual can be and often is a glib talker and an outgoing person, provided the failure of academic life has not taken too heavy a toll.

While the mildly dislexic individual may be thought of as nothing more than an otherwise bright, but careless student, the more severely dyslexic may be labeled as dull, recalcitrant, delinquent, or even retarded. As dyslexia becomes more severe, the problems with reading increase. Since there is no rule that one who is dyslexic must have a high IQ to offset the reading problem, a cruel twist of fate can occur where a child has both dyslexia and a borderline IQ.

Physical difficulties may also occur. We have such a patient who in addition to having severe dyslexia has bilateral optic atrophy, which occurred after childhood meningitis. The best visual acuity is 20/80, but because of the overlying dyslexia, which was backed up with a very strong family history, the child was 12 years old before proper interpretation of the organic visual difficulty could be made. When physical problems are combined with the obvious problems of primary specific developmental dyslexia, an individual is indeed handicapped and especially in need of thorough and accurate psychological testing to determine the level of intelligence. This, of course, is outside the expertise of the ophthalmologist.

EYE EXAMINATION IN THE SUSPECTED DYSLEXIC INDIVIDUAL

The eye examination done on a suspected dyslexic child consists of a routine eye examination, with a few additional procedures.

Paragraph reading

Children are asked to read a standard paragraph of J-2 sized print. This paragraph is excerpted from Benjamin Franklin's autobiography. The J-2 paragraph begins "I walked up the street, gazing about until near the market house I spied a boy with bread. I had made many a meal on bread and asked him where he got it. . . ." After listening to hundreds of children of all types read this paragraph, several patterns have emerged.

1. Young children who are good readers read fluently until they come to an unfamiliar word. At this time, they slow down to sound out the unfamiliar word and in most instances either get the word or come close. In the first sentence, "gazing" and "market house" are such words.

2. Poor readers with exogenous dyslexia or lack of educational stimulation or patients with a low IQ stop completely when they come to a word they do

not know and will not proceed. Depending on age and ability, such children stop sooner or later in the paragraph. There is little tendency on the part of such children to sound out words or to skip ahead to arrive at a meaning for the sentence or paragraph. This slow, stubborn behavior can be exasperating in the examining room and must be even more so in the classroom.

3. Dyslexic students, on the other hand, have a unique response to this paragraph reading. They skip over words they have difficulty with while attempting to make some sense out of the material read. An otherwise bright dyslexic child might read the illustrative paragraph as follows: "I *went* (walked) up the street, *going* (gazing) *around* (about) until near the — pause — market*place* (house) I *saw* (met) a boy with bread (no pause for the period) I . . . ." This paragraph has been extremely valuable to us in the evaluation of dyslexia.

Comprehension and visual-motor performance

In addition to paragraph reading, the workup for the suspected dyslexic patient continues as follows:

PLATE 14-1

A The child is asked to draw a man. No further instructions are given. He may make the figure as small or as large as he wants, as detailed or as simple.

B The examiner draws a circle approximately 2 inches in diameter and asks the child to fill in the face of a clock, with the hands indicating that the time is 3 o'clock.

C The child is asked to draw a bicycle.

D The child is asked to print or write his name, depending on the type of writing that is being done in school.

E The patient is asked to copy geometric figures, which include drawing a square in an already drawn triangle and to draw a diamond in an already drawn square.

As with the interpretation of paragraph reading, the information to be gained from evaluation of the above drawing and writing is highly subjective. However, with experience and patience, the ophthalmologist can get some idea as to how adept the child is at carrying out the above tasks. For example, if the child has no concept of filling the space while drawing the clock and crowds all of the numbers over to one side, it is possible that some type of soft neurologic deficit may exist. Also, immature children with low intelligence in general do a sloppier job on all the tasks. Since parents and often teachers are very much taken with the concept of "eye-hand coordination," asking the patient to carry out certain drawing activities confirms an awareness of the importance of fine motor activities on the part of the ophthalmologist. Poor performance in this area certainly seems a logical basis for suggesting pediatric neurologic evaluation in appropriate cases since the tasks are also a measure of parietal lobe function.

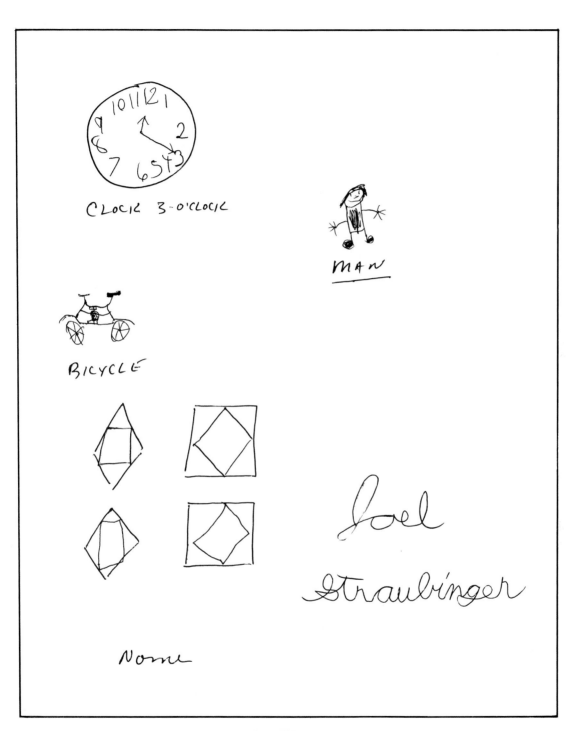

CLOCK 3-O'CLOCK

MAN

BICYCLE

Joel
Straubinger

Name

PLATE 14-1

Eye function and dyslexia

The examination, including paragraph reading and drawing and writing exercises, is always done in the presence of the family and the interpretation is shared with them. Actually, the child's performance with these tasks may help the family understand some of the subtle possibilities regarding a neurologic basis for dyslexia. This is especially so when, as in most cases, the ophthalmologist has demonstrated that the child has 20/20 vision and normal stereopsis, normal ocular motility, and so on. At the conclusion of the eye examination, it is important to convey to the family a sincere interest in the child and his or her academic problem. Merely saying that the eyes have nothing to do with reading failure and then ushering the patient and family out breeds hostility and frustration and will encourage the family to seek out one of the practicioners who is willing to "at least try something." Often these individuals provide expensive, time-consuming, and sometimes harmful activities for these children. Since the eyes are an essential intermediary between the printed page and the human brain, some response to the question "what is the role of eye function in reading disability?" is unavoidable. For this reason, it is sometimes necessary to reassure parents and others by explaining the specific role of various eye functions in learning disability.

Specific eye functions as they relate to reading ability and dyslexia may be characterized as follows:

Visual acuity

An individual cannot read ordinary print without sight (although he or she may read Braille). However, even with poor sight correctable to 20/200 or less (which is legal blindness), some motivated individuals can read. They read more slowly than a normally sighted individual but with comprehension at their level of intelligence. Visual acuity and dyslexia are not related.

Refractive error

The need for glasses, when properly met with spectacles or contact lenses, has no significant effect on reading ability and is not related to dyslexia. So-called training lenses have no beneficial effect on reading ability and may produce a harmful dependence if improperly prescribed. Many myopic or nearsighted children are actually better readers then comparable children without need for glasses.

Eye muscle imbalance

Crossing of the eyes is significant only when a latent in-turning or out-drifting of the eyes is present that causes serious eye fatigue and discomfort while reading. This eye fatigue can lead to poor reading performance and a lack of enthusiasm for reading. Correction of these conditions with surgery, lenses, prisms, or exercises—whichever is appropriate—can lead to improved reading performance. Eye muscle imbalance in any of its manifestations is unrelated to the decoding process and therefore is not related to true dyslexia.

Color vision

The ability to recognize and name most colors is unrelated to reading performance or dyslexia. On the other hand, a total absence of color vision (congenital achromatopia) is a rare and serious eye defect associated with legal blindness (20/200 corrected vision). This is not to be confused with the mild red-green color defect that affects 8% of men and less than 1% of women. Blue-yellow color blindness is extremely rare. (The inability to read ditto sheets is probably related to poor reproduction — not to an inability to discern the blue color.)

Fusion ability

The ability to superimpose and blend the visual image from each eye unless it causes a latent muscle imbalance has no influence on reading ability.

Accommodation

This is the process of increasing the dioptric power of the eye as objects are brought nearer to the eye (also called focusing ability). When this reflex is sluggish or hypoactive, difficulty in reading can occur. This condition is rare and is treated with specific eye drops or with bifocals. Empirically prescribed bifocals supposedly for general improvement of scholastic performance have no beneficial effect on reading ability and may, if worn for a long period, produce rather than help hypoaccommodation. Hypoaccommodation can cause slow reading but is not a cause of dyslexia.

Dominant eye

This is the sighting eye or the eye preferred under monocular circumstances. It has been found to have no relationship to reading ability or dyslexia.

Controlling eye

This is the eye preferred under binocular conditions. It has no relationship to reading ability or dyslexia.

Pursuit movements

The ability of the eyes to follow a test object smoothly or to progress in smooth steps across a printed page has no causal relationship to poor reading. On the other hand, a poor reader often has jerky and frequent refixations while reading across a line or down a page. This is a result rather than a cause of poor reading. No relationship exists between the ability of the eyes to perform pursuit movements and dyslexia.

Perception or cerebral processing

This rather elusive and multifactorial process takes place at higher cortical levels and takes into consideration many factors, not the least of which is experience. The eyes merely provide neural impulses to the brain. The brain, in turn, perceives and makes intellectual judgments with regard to the impulses provided. Dyslexia may be a type of imperception or misperception, but the defect occurs centrally in the brain and is not caused by peripheral nervous system involvement or eye malfunction.

Eye-hand-body coordination

This refers to how the hand or body relates to and acts upon what is perceived by the brain. Clumsiness or poor body coordination has been treated extensively at times even by individuals whose formal training and usual activities are ordinarily related to the eye. These practicioners have been known to instruct patients in such activities as drawing circles, walking on a balance board, and following objects with their eyes. A certain group has even instructed children in assuming certain positions during sleep in the hope a "neurologic reorientation" will take place that will cause them to function in a more normal way upon awakening. These activities have no beneficial effect on the eyes, are not in the province of the ophthalmologist, have been shown by most experts to have no effect upon reading, and may even be harmful.

What then is the role of the ophthalmologist in this problem of reading disability in general and dyslexia in particular? The answer is: He or she must care for the eyes in a carefully planned preventive program of visual and eye care; when specific needs arise he or she must treat any disease or malfunction that occurs. To do this, vision should be tested beginning in the preschool years (between the third and fourth birthday), and glasses and other appropriate treatment should be prescribed only when needed. When eye muscle imbalance is found, it should be treated. While treatment is being carried out, the use of glasses, prisms, eye drops, exercises, and in some cases surgery, should be available to the physician and the patient when necessary. The eye physician should cooperate with the educator and assist as a member of an interdisciplinary team that includes such specialties as neurology, pediatrics, audiology, psychiatry, psychology, social work, and education. The ophthalmologist should protect the patient and his or her family from the frequently recurring useless and sometimes harmful fads promoted by those who would exploit the role of the eyes in reading for reasons of ignorance or profit.

288

BIBLIOGRAPHY

The following is a list of books and articles that contain additional information on subjects introduced in this book. Our purpose is to provide the reader of *Pediatric ophthalmology practice* with a problem-solving tool while at the same time encouraging him to consult more detailed sources of information in areas that are beyond the scope of this book.

1. Beard, C.: Ptosis, St. Louis, ed. 2, 1976, The C. V. Mosby Co.
2. Breuggeman, W. G., and Helveston, E. M.: Ketamine, Ophthalmic Surg. **2**(6): 243-245, 1971.
3. Critchley, M.: Developmental dyslexia, London, 1964, William Heineman Medical Books.
4. Ellis, F. D., and Helveston, E. M., editors: Strabismus surgery, International Ophthalmology Clinics, **16**(3), Boston, Fall 1976, Little, Brown and Co.
5. Ellis, F. D., and Yune, H. Y.: Optic nerve anomaly, midline facial anomaly and basal encephalocele, Perspect. Ophthalmol. **2**(1):43-48, 1978.
6. Ellsworth, R.: Retinoblastoma. In Duane, T., editor, Clinical ophthalmology, ch. 35, New York, 1976, Harper & Row, Publishers.
7. Faye, E. E.: Clinical low vision, Boston, 1976, Little, Brown and Co.
8. Flynn, J. T., Acute proliferative retrolental fibroplasia: evolution of the lescon, Albrecht von Graefes Arch. Klen. Ophthalmol. **195**:101, 1975.
9. Francois, J.: Congenital cataracts, Assen, Netherlands, 1963, Charles C Thomas, Publisher, Royal Van Gorcum Publishers.
10. Gay, A. J., Newman, N. M., Keltner, J. L., and Stroud, M. H.: Eye movement disorders, St. Louis, 1974, The C. V. Mosby Co.
11. Goldberg, M. F., editor: Genetic and metabolic eye disease, Boston, 1974, Little, Brown and Co.
12. Goldberg, H. K., and Schiffman, G.: Dyslexia problems of reading disabilities, New York, 1972, Grune & Stratton, Inc.
13. Goodman, R. M., and Gorlin, R. J.: Atlas of the face in genetic disorders, ed. 2, St. Louis, 1977, The C. V. Mosby Co.

14. Grant, W. M., and Walton, D. S.: Progressive changes in the angle in congenital aniridia, with development of glaucoma, Am. J. Ophthalmol. **78**(5):842-847, Nov. 1974.
15. Grayson, M.: Diseases of the cornea, St. Louis, 1979, The C. V. Mosby Co.
16. Harley, R. D., editor: Pediatric Ophthalmology, Philadelphia, 1975, W. B. Saunders Co.
17. Hartstein, J., editor: Current concepts in dyslexia, St. Louis, 1971, The C. V. Mosby Co.
18. Helveston, E. M.: Atlas of strabismus surgery, ed. 2, St. Louis, 1977, The C. V. Mosby Co.
19. Helveston, E. M., and Biglan, A. W.: Retinoblastoma: a ten-year experience with a regional treatment center, Perspect. Ophthalmol. **2**(1):27-34, March 1978.
20. Hiles, D. A., editor: Infantile cataract surgery, International Ophthalmology Clinics, **17**(14), Boston, 1977, Little, Brown and Co.
21. Jones, L. T., and Wobig, J. L.: Surgery of the eyelids and lacrimal system, Birmingham, 1976, Aesculopius Publishing Co.
22. Keeney, A. H., and Keeney, V. T., editors: Dyslexia, St. Louis, 1968, The C. V. Mosby Co.
23. Kennedy, R. E.: The effect of early enucleation on the orbit, Am. J. Ophthalmol. **60**:227, 1965.
24. Kolkar, A. E., and Hetherington, J., Jr.: Becker-Shaffer's diagnosis and therapy of the glaucomas, ed. 4, St. Louis, 1976, The C. V. Mosby Co.
25. Krill, A. E.: Hereditary retinal and choroidal diseases, vol. I, Hagerstown, 1972, Harper & Row, Publishers.
26. Krill, A. E., and Archer, D. B.: Krill's hereditary retinal and choroidal diseases, vol. II, Hagerstown, Md., 1977, Harper & Row, Publishers.
27. Kreshner, B. J., Essner, D., Cohen, I. J., and Flynn, J. T.: Retrolental fibroplasia: II, pathologic correlation, Arch. Ophthalmol. **95**:29, 1977.
28. Kwitko, M. L., editor: Surgery of the infant eye, New York, 1979, Appleton-Century-Crofts.
29. Liebman, S. D., and Gellis, S. S., editors: The pediatrician's ophthalmology, St. Louis, 1966, The C. V. Mosby Co.
30. Link, A.: On writing, reading and dyslexia, New York, 1973, Grune & Stratton, Inc.
31. McCormick, A. Q.: Current problems in pediatrics, retinopathy of prematurity, **7**(11), Chicago, 1977, Year Book Medical Publishers, Inc.
32. Mustarde, J. C., Jones, L. T., and Callahan, A.: Ophthalmic plastic surgery — up-to-date, Birmingham, 1970, Aesculopius Publishing Co.
33. Noorden, G. K. von: Burian — von Noorden's binocular vision and ocular motility, ed. 2, St. Louis, 1979, The C. V. Mosby Co.
34. Noorden, G. K. von: von Noorden-Maumenee's Atlas of strabismus, ed. 3, St. Louis, 1977, The C. V. Mosby Co.
35. Ophthalmology basic and clinical science course, continuing education in ophthalmology, section 1-10, American Academy of Ophthalmology, San Francisco, 1979-1980.
36. Ophthalmologic staff of the Hospital for Sick Children, Toronto: The eye in childhood, Chicago, 1967, Year Book Medical Publishers, Inc.
37. Parks, M. M.: Ocular motility and strabismus, Hagerstown, Md., 1975, Harper & Row, Publishers.
38. Roth, A. M.: Retinal vasculature development in premature infants, Arch. Ophthalmol. **84**(5): 636, 1977.

39. Rubin, M. L.: Optics for clinicians, Gainesville, Fla., 1971, Tread Scientific Publishers.
40. Schlaegel, T. F.: Essentials of uveitis, Boston, 1969, Little, Brown and Co.
41. Shaffer, R. N., and Hoskins, H. D., Jr.: Congenital glaucomas CETV, Ophth. Am. Acad. Ophthalmol. and Otolarygol. Oph 4 Vol. III, 1977.
42. Shaffer, R. N., and Weiss, D. I.: Congenital and pediatric glaucomas, St. Louis, 1970, The C. V. Mosby Co.
43. Tasman, W., editor: Retinal diseases in children, New York, 1971, Harper & Row, Publishers.
44. Terry, T. L.: Extreme prematurity and fibroblastic overgrowth of persistent vascular sheath behind each crystalline lens: preliminary report, Am. J. Ophthalmol. **25:**203, 1942.
45. Tessier, P.: Total facial osteotomies for correction of the syndromes of Crouzon and Apert, oxycephalies and scaphocephalies, **42:**501, 1968.
46. Wilson, W. A.: Cataracts and guloctose metabolism, Tr. Am. Ophthalmol. Soc. **65:**661, 1967.
47. Worst, J. G. F.: The pathogenesis of congenital glaucoma, Assen, Netherlands, 1966, Charles C Thomas, Publisher, Royal Van Gorcum Publishers.

INDEX